Building Tissues

An Engineer's Guide to Regenerative Medicine

Biomedical Engineering Series

Donald R. Peterson, Series Editor

Published Titles

Electromagnetic Analysis and Design in Magnetic Resonance Imaging,
Jianming Jin

Endogenous and Exogenous Regulation and Control of Physiological Systems,
Robert B. Northrop

Artificial Neural Networks in Cancer Diagnosis, Prognosis, and Treatment,
Raouf N.G. Naguib and Gajanan V. Sherbet

Medical Image Registration,
Joseph V. Hajnal, Derek Hill, and David J. Hawkes

Introduction to Dynamic Modeling of Neuro-Sensory Systems,
Robert B. Northrop

Noninvasive Instrumentation and Measurement in Medical Diagnosis,
Robert B. Northrop

Handbook of Neuroprosthetic Methods,
Warren E. Finn and Peter G. LoPresti

Angiography and Plaque Imaging: Advanced Segmentation Techniques,
Jasjit S. Suri and Swamy Laxminarayan

Biomedical Image Analysis,
Rangaraj M. Rangayyan

Foot and Ankle Motion Analysis: Clinical Treatment and Technology,
Gerald F. Harris, Peter A. Smith, Richard M. Marks

Introduction to Molecular Biology, Genomics and Proteomic for Biomedical Engineers,
Robert B. Northrop and Anne N. Connor

Signals and Systems Analysis in Biomedical Engineering, Second Edition,
Robert B. Northrop

An Introduction to Biomaterials, Second Edition,
Jeffrey O. Hollinger

Analysis and Application of Analog Electronic Circuits to Biomedical Instrumentation, Second Edition,
Robert B. Northrop

Non-Invasive Instrumentation and Measurement in Medical Diagnosis,
Robert B. Northrop

Building Tissues: An Engineer's Guide to Regenerative Medicine,
Joseph W. Freeman, Debabrata Banerjee

Please visit our website www.crcpress.com for a full list of titles

Building Tissues

An Engineer's Guide to Regenerative Medicine

Joseph W. Freeman

Debabrata Banerjee

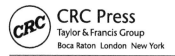

CRC Press
Taylor & Francis Group
Boca Raton London New York

CRC Press is an imprint of the
Taylor & Francis Group, an **Informa** business

First published in paperback 2024

First published 2019
by CRC Press
2385 NW Executive Center Drive, Suite 320, Boca Raton FL 33431

and by CRC Press
4 Park Square, Milton Park, Abingdon, Oxon, OX14 4RN

CRC Press is an imprint of Taylor & Francis Group, LLC

No claim to original U.S. Government works

© 2019, 2024 Taylor & Francis Group, LLC

ISBN: 978-1-4987-4280-1 (hbk)
ISBN: 978-1-03-265233-7 (pbk)
ISBN: 978-0-429-42902-6 (ebk)

DOI: 10.1201/9780429429026

Visit the Taylor & Francis Web site at
http://www.taylorandfrancis.com

and the CRC Press Web site at
http://www.crcpress.com

Contents

Preface

BIOMEDICAL ENGINEERING IS A unique area in engineering because it combines classical engineering principles (from chemical, mechanical, and electrical engineering) with aspects of biology. In most biomedical engineering applications, the engineering aspect is the major force behind the technology, which then interacts with biological systems. This is seen in neural implants (electrical engineering), metallic implants (mechanical engineering), drug-delivery systems (chemical engineering), and other technologies. One area where this is not necessarily the case is tissue engineering. In tissue engineering, there is a major focus on biology because we are essentially growing tissue as seen in nature. To develop tissues, we take cues from natural development, using concepts from biology including cellular biology, cell signaling, extracellular matrix production, biocompatibility, and bioactivity. The overwhelming importance of these concepts can sometimes make engineering concepts seem unimportant. There are many high-quality important manuscripts in tissue engineering that do not explicitly discuss many of the mathematical concepts that are typically ascribed to engineering. Although they are not always spelled out explicitly in the literature, these principles are still present. After all, the human body is a machine, and machine performance is based on engineering concepts.

Musculoskeletal tissues operate under tensile, compressive, and shear stresses, which lead to complementary strains in their matrices. Scaffolds used to replace these tissues must have comparable moduli and ultimate stresses. The cells within these tissues experience these stresses and strains and respond to them in various ways. When seeding cells into a scaffold, tissue engineers are concerned about the transfer of oxygen and nutrients to the cells and the removal of waste products from the cells; this is a form of mass transfer. In addition, tissue engineering involves aspects of material science. Tissue engineers must know what materials are available to them, what are the criteria for material selection, and how to select the best material for the task. Once the material is selected, new questions arise: What type of scaffold structure is needed? What techniques can give you the properties necessary for success?

These engineering questions in combination with biological considerations must be taken into account. What cell type is best for this application? How do I best stimulate these cells for tissue development? What are the limitations of the chosen method for stimulating cell proliferation and differentiation? How does the chosen cell type interact with certain materials?

This book brings both of these worlds together to develop the next generation of competent tissue engineers with a balanced knowledge base in both engineering and biology. It provides basic engineering and biological concepts in a way that relates to tissue function and tissue engineering. We discuss tissue function beginning at the molecular level and continuing to the entire tissue. Readers will learn about the importance of material composition and internal architecture in the function of complex tissues. These concepts are then carried into an introduction to tissue mechanics and behavior where readers are given examples of how engineering concepts are present in the everyday function of tissues and engineered replacements. The text also gives the reader options for replacement and cellular scaffolds, including materials and scaffolding structures. We also discuss the available options for cells to initiate the production of the regenerated tissue. What cells are best for which application and how to stimulate them for the ultimate goal of tissue regeneration?

It is our hope that this text will be a step in bridging this gap, providing students with ways to apply basic engineering to biology and giving engineers basic biology that can be applied to tissue engineering.

Joseph W. Freeman

Acknowledgments

THIS BOOK REQUIRED THE work and support of several individuals. I would like to thank my work study students Joscandy Nunez and Benton Cheng for their contributions. I would also like to thank Michael Slaughter for encouraging me to take on this project.

Authors

Joseph W. Freeman is an associate professor in the Department of Biomedical Engineering at Rutgers University. He has worked in the areas of tendon development, the structure and mechanics of type I collagen, collagen mineralization and mechanical characterization, molecular modeling, soft tissue mechanics, and musculoskeletal tissue engineering. His primary research focus now lies in the design and fabrication of novel, functional scaffolds for the repair of musculoskeletal tissues, the fabrication and use of novel biomaterials in tissue regeneration, developing therapies for tissue strengthening, and the use of tissue engineering techniques in cancer research. He has published numerous papers in a variety of scientific journals and delivered seminars, invited talks, and conference presentations in these areas. He has taught the courses in tissue engineering, transport, mechanics of materials, biomechanics.

Debabrata Banerjee is an associate professor in the Department of Pharmacology at the Robert Wood Johnson Medical Center. He has been an active researcher in tissue engineering and now stem cell technologies for the past 12 years. His focus is on molecular mechanisms that use stem cells, which are proving to be highly beneficial to tissue regeneration. He has published more than 150 papers in tissue engineering and regenerative medicine journals.

CHAPTER 1

Stress and Strain Analyses

1.1 INTRODUCTION

Your body is subjected to a multitude of forces with every step, every breath, and every heartbeat. A variety of forces can produce different effects on different tissues. When these forces are applied to tissues, they produce stresses and strains. Tendons and ligaments are stretched, bones are compressed, blood shears the inner surfaces of blood vessels and stretches their walls. To function correctly, specific tissues must be able to withstand certain forces. A tissue engineer must be aware of these forces and produce scaffolds that can withstand them when they are implanted. In this section we will introduce the reader to the concepts of force, stress, and strain. For a more in-depth analysis of these topics the reader may want to read *Mechanics of Materials* by Ferdinand P. Beer, E. Russell Johnston, Jr., and John T. DeWolf or *Engineering Mechanics: Statics* by J. L. Meriam and L. G. Kraige.[1,2] Both of these texts were used as references for this section.

1.2 CALCULATING FORCES

These forces are applied in different directions and in different ways. The most commonly studied are normal forces. These forces act perpendicular to the planes that they are affecting and create normal stresses on the object that they are placed on. In this chapter we will review how to solve for the magnitude of forces and use the forces to calculate normal stresses. We will then review how these stresses affect objects through changes in the objects' lengths.

One way to calculate the magnitude of the force acting on an object is to use statics. We will perform a quick review of statics and use it to solve for the forces acting on the tissues in a basic biomechanics problem. Statics allows us to calculate the magnitude of the forces placed on an object through a series of equilibrium balances. For example, we have the following situation:

PROBLEM 1.1

A person is carrying a purse from their forearm (at the elbow) as seen in Figure 1.1. The purse is really packed and weighs 40 Newtons (40 N). We want to calculate the forces at the elbow and the places where the bicep is connected to the bone. We can model this system using the following set of figures.

In Figure 1.1b, we have modeled the arm and purse. The upper arm is the striped bar, the forearm is the white bar, and the biceps muscle is the solid black bar. The muscle is connected to the forearm and upper arm by tendons. The forearm has a 40-N bag hanging off of it. To simplify things, we have neglected the weight of the hand and remainder of the forearm, so the forearm is cutoff at the point where the bag hangs. We want to know the forces being placed onto the elbow and the tendon, points A and B, seen in Figure 1.1c. The force from the bag is going to lead to forces at points A and B, as seen in Figure 1.1d. To simplify the problem, we will say that the weight of the forearm is negligible. The length between A and B is 23 cm. The tendon forms an angle of 83.8° with the forearm. We notice that the object is not moving. Therefore, the object is in equilibrium and the problem can be solved by using statics. The first thing we do is write a balance equation for the forces in the x and y directions.

$$\sum F_x = 0 = A_x + T_x$$

$$A_x = -T_x$$

$$\sum F_y = 0 = A_y + T_y - 40\text{N} = 0$$

$$A_y + T_y = 40\text{N}$$

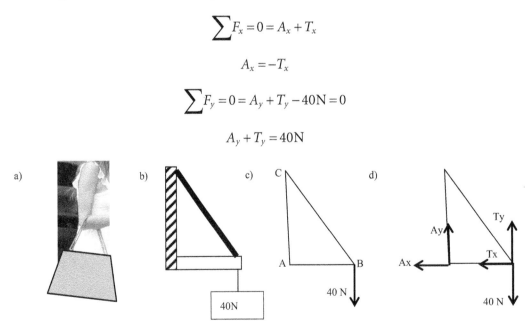

FIGURE 1.1 This figure shows the transformation of a load bearing situation into a free body diagram. (a) Picture of someone holding a purse. (b) A diagram representing the purse as a weight acting on the bottom portion of a hinge joint. (c) A free body diagram representing the purse as a weight acting at a point on the forearm. (d) The full free body diagram with the weight of the lures and reaction forces at the elbow (hinge joint).

Note the signs in the force balance in the y direction. The 40 N from the bag is negative because it is acting downward in the negative y direction. To balance this force, T_y and C_y are acting upward in the positive y direction.

To find the magnitudes of A_y and T_y, we need an additional balance. We will use a moment balance for our last equation. A moment is the distance between a point A and the point where a force has been applied (point B) multiplied by the magnitude of the portion of the force that is perpendicular to the line of the distance, $\overline{AB}$. The distance $\overline{AB}$ is called the *moment arm*.

In this case, we will take the sum of the moments about point A. For the force T_y, our moment arm is the distance between points A and B. For the 40 N force from the bag, our moment arm is also the distance between points A and B.

$$\sum M_A = T_y\left(\overline{AB}\right) - (40N)\left(\overline{AB}\right) = 0$$

Note that the forces at point A_x and A_y are not in the equation. These forces pass through point A, so their moment arms have lengths of zero. If this equation is true, then T_y is 40 N. This means that according to the previous equation:

$$A_y + T_y = 40N$$

$$\therefore A_y = 0$$

Now that we know the value of T_y we can solve for T_x and also T.

$$T_y = T\sin 83.8 = 40N$$

$$T = \frac{40N}{\sin 83.8} = 40.24N$$

Now we know how the bag affects forces at the joint and the tendon. So if we were designing a replacement tendon or muscle, we would have to make sure that it could withstand these forces to prevent failure.

1.3 CALCULATING STRESSES

To compare the results of forces on different materials with different shapes, engineers typically normalize the forces by dividing them by the areas upon which they act. This yields a stress; a stress is defined as force per unit area (F/A). Its units are Pascals (Pa) in the SI metric system and pounds per square inch (psi) in the US system.

We can apply this to the previous problem by dividing the calculated forces at B and C with the cross-sectional area for biceps tendons. We now know the forces that the tendon would be subjected to and divide them by the areas that they are acting on. Because these forces are pulling on the tendon, they are tensile, and we will be using the cross-sectional areas of the tendons. The biceps tendon diameters range from around 5 to 6 mm,[3,4] we will use 5.5 mm as our diameter. Modeling a circular cross-section, the area of the tendons in the problem is 23.8 mm². Dividing this by the force in the muscle-tendon unit (40.23 N), we obtain a stress of 1.69×10^6 Pa or 1.69 Megapascals (MPa).

Based on these calculations, our tendon replacement must be able to withstand a stress of 1.69 MPa. So, the combination of the material and scaffolding technique must produce a structure that can withstand this stress without failure or displaying signs of fatigue.

You may be asking yourself, but why use stress? If you calculate a force shouldn't that be enough to tell you what is going on with your scaffold or the cells on the scaffold? Stress tells you how the force is applied and the potential effect it can have on a material, device, organism, and more. For example, let's say you are watering a plant with a hose. The water is coming out of the hose at a low flow rate and travels a certain distance horizontally away from the hose. If you put your hand in the stream of water, it does not hurt at all. Now you decide to put your thumb over half of the opening of the hose. What happens? The water comes out of the hose more forcefully. It travels horizontally away from the hose a further distance. If you put your hand under the stream, it may sting a little. What happened? How did you get such different effects from water running through the same hose? The answer is stress. A certain amount of water was moving through the opening of the hose every second. When you place your thumb over the hose, you cut down on the shape of the opening and you decrease its area. What about the water? Because the hose didn't swell with backed up water, the same amount of water is traveling through the hose as before. Cutting the area of the opening increased the pressure created by the water.

PROBLEM 1.2

Let's apply the concept of stress in a more practical way. We will see the importance of stress by looking at footwear. A 200-lb man is walking and steps on your foot with the heel of his sneaker. Let's say the heel of the sneaker has a total area of 27 cm². We will estimate that half of his weight is on your foot. So that is 100 pounds or about 90 kg. To turn this mass into a force, we must multiply it by the acceleration due to gravity (9.8 m/s²). This gives us 882 kg• m/s² or 882 N. It comes down on a section of your foot that is 27 cm², so the stress is 882/27, which gives us 32.6×10^4 N/m or 326 kPa (kilopascals). When he steps on your foot it hurts briefly, but you are fine.

Later you and that same man go to a costume party. You dress up as a surfer wearing sandals and he decides to dress up as a woman and is wearing high-heeled shoes. He steps on your foot again, but this time you scream and fall to the floor. Why was it so painful this time as opposed to last time? Once again, it comes down to the stress. Let's say that the heel of the shoe as an area of 3 cm² or 3×10^{-4} m². When you divide half of his weight by this number you get 2.94×10^6 Pa $\approx$ 3MPa (Megapascals). The amount of stress increases by almost 10 times. Let's look at the math (Figure 1.2).

So stress is very important. It determines how a material, tissue, scaffold, and more will react to an applied force.

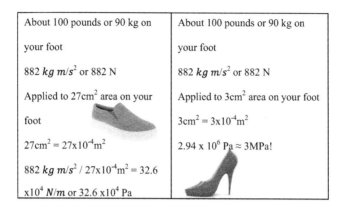

About 100 pounds or 90 kg on your foot	About 100 pounds or 90 kg on your foot
$882\ kg\ m/s^2$ or 882 N	$882\ kg\ m/s^2$ or 882 N
Applied to 27cm^2 area on your foot	Applied to 3cm^2 area on your foot
$27cm^2 = 27 \times 10^{-4} m^2$	$3cm^2 = 3 \times 10^{-4} m^2$
$882\ kg\ m/s^2 / 27 \times 10^{-4} m^2 = 32.6 \times 10^4\ N/m$ or 32.6×10^4 Pa	2.94×10^6 Pa $\approx$ 3MPa!

FIGURE 1.2   Calculations of the stress produced when wearing a flat shoe or a high-heeled shoe.

1.3.1 Normal Stresses

Now that we can solve for forces, we can use them to solve for stresses. As discussed, stress is defined as the force per unit area (F/A). There are several different types of stress; the differences lie in where and how the force is applied.

Normal stresses are caused by forces that act perpendicular to a surface. Normal stresses can be tensile or compressive (Figure 1.3). Tensile stresses occur when you have two forces acting on an object from different directions along the same axis. This causes stretching of the object. When the two forces are acting toward each other along the same axis, this creates compression, where the object is being crushed by the two forces.

The magnitude of a normal stress can be found using the following equation:

$$\sigma = \frac{P}{A}$$

Where σ is the stress, P is the force, and A is the area of the surface that the force is acting on. If the stress creates tension, it has a positive sign; if it creates compression, it has a negative sign. Normal stresses are common in orthopedics. Ligaments and tendons operate primarily under tension during everyday use. The two previous problems are examples of this. Their collagen fibers are aligned mainly down the long axis to provide them with more strength in this direction. Therefore, tissue engineers must be conscious of the tensile forces placed on these tissues *in vivo* and must be sure that their scaffold or the tissue that they have developed in the bioreactor can withstand these stresses once implanted.

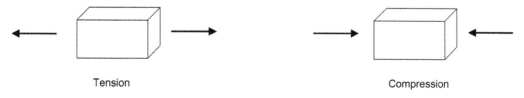

Tension   Compression

FIGURE 1.3   Examples of tension and compression.

PROBLEM 1.3

After a traumatic accident, an actor has just had his deltoid tendon replaced by a tissue-engineered scaffold developed by your company. After surgery, the implant is working well, but it has not been placed under a large amount of load yet. The actor has recently been offered a role in a medieval movie as a sword-wielding knight. His doctor gives you a call because she wants to know if the implant will be able to stand up the stresses of holding a sword in this movie. Knowing the mechanics of the implant and looking through the information on the patient, you run some quick preliminary calculations to put the doctor and patient at ease. You need to find the force on the deltoid tendon, convert that into a tensile stress, and then compare that to the ultimate tensile stress of the implant.

Your implant has a cross-sectional area of 5 cm^2 and an ultimate tensile stress of 35 MPa. You have been told that the actor's sword weighs 6 N. He will hold the sword upright at the center of mass of his hand. The deltoid tendon forms an angle of 15° with the humerus and attaches at a point on the humerus 0.14 m away from the shoulder. The other lengths are:

0.60 m from shoulder to the force from the hand.

0.35 m from shoulder to the force from the forearm.

0.15 m from shoulder to the force from the upper arm (Figure 1.4).

When the actor is just holding the sword (not swinging it), the most force will be placed on the implant when the sword is being held in an outstretched arm (largest moment arm). Therefore, we will use this position for our calculations. We can split the arm into sections,

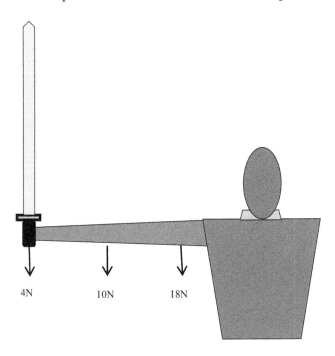

FIGURE 1.4   Schematic of actor holding sword.

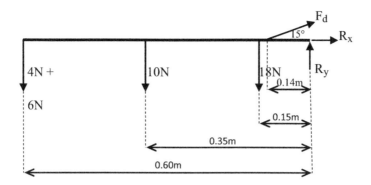

FIGURE 1.5   Free body diagram of actor holding the sword.

each with its own weight. To find the force placed on the deltoid tendon, we will once again use statics; as part of this method, we assume the loading situation is in equilibrium. This means that the sum of all forces along the axes equal zero, and the sum of all of the moments about each axis equals zero. We will use these facts to write three equilibrium balances.

First we draw a free body diagram to look at all of the forces (Figure 1.5). Then we write out our equilibrium balances based on the diagram.

$$\sum F_x = F_d \cos\theta + R_x = 0$$

$$\sum F_y = F_d \sin\theta + R_y - W_{H+S} - W_F - W_U = 0$$

$$\sum M = W_{H+S}r_H + W_F r_F + W_U r_U - F_d r_d \sin\theta = 0$$

To solve for the force in the deltoid tendon, F_d, we only need to use the sum of the moments equation.

$$\sum M = (10\text{N})(0.6\,\text{m}) + (10\text{N})(0.35\,\text{m}) + (18\text{N})(0.15\,\text{m}) = F_d(0.14\,\text{m})\sin 15°$$

$$6\,N\text{m} + 3.5\,N\text{m} + 2.7\,N\text{m} = (0.036\,\text{m})F_d$$

$$338.89\,\text{N} = F_d$$

To tear the implant the stress must exceed the ultimate tensile stress 35 MPa

$$\sigma = \frac{F}{A} = \frac{338.89}{0.05\,\text{m}^2} = 6,777.8 \text{ Pa or } 6.78 \text{ kPa}$$

Because 6.78 kPa is far less than 35 MPa, the implant is will not fail from holding the sword.

Compressive stresses are a major concern in bone and cartilage tissue engineering. Bone is designed to withstand large compressive loads, and articular cartilage (hyaline cartilage)

Diameter = 10 mm

Outer
diameter = 10 mm

FIGURE 1.6   Scaffolds for bone tissue engineering.

is designed to absorb the shock of compressive loads. Engineers must design bone scaffolds with enough stiffness to withstand these forces without failing. This is particularly important for the long bones in the leg. Scaffolds for cartilage must resist failure under compressive loads while remaining compliant. This is especially important in the knees.

PROBLEM 1.4

You have built a porous, mineralized scaffold to regenerate new bone. You have tested for biocompatibility, and it has fared well. Now you want to test its mechanical strength (Figure 1.6).

You apply a force of 1,000 N onto the scaffold with dimensions shown given here. What is the stress experienced by the sample? This is a simple calculation; we just divide the force by the cross-sectional area, πr^2. When the scaffold has a hole in the center, the area changes to the area of the outer shape minus the area of the inner shape (the hole).

So the stress placed on the first implant is:

$$\frac{1000 \text{N}}{(\pi)5 \text{mm}^2} = 12.73 \text{MPa}$$

The stress placed on the second implant:

$$\frac{1000 \text{N}}{\left((\pi)5^2\right) - \left((\pi)2.5^2\right)} = 16.98 \text{MPa}$$

So the decrease in area (because of the hole) causes an increase in the stress placed on the implant, and on the cells seeded onto the implant.

1.4 DEFORMATION AND STRAIN

An applied force or stress results in a change in the length of an object. For smaller forces or stresses, this change can be extremely small; for larger forces, the change can lead to complete failure. This change in length is called a *deformation*. The deformation from a normal force is given by the following equation:

$$\delta = \frac{PL}{EA}$$

where δ is the change in length, *P* is the applied force, *L* is the distance from the applied force to the base, *E* is the elastic modulus of the material (a measure of strength that will be discussed later), and *A* is the cross-sectional area over which the force is applied.

PROBLEM 1.5

You are evaluating the design of the new load-bearing scaffolds for bone replacement used in Problem 1.4. Using the same loading conditions, how much is each implant compressed? Both implants have heights of 20 mm and elastic moduli, *E*, of 2 GPa

For the first implant:

$$\delta = \frac{(1000\,\text{N})(20\,\text{mm})}{(2\,\text{GPa})(\pi)(5\,\text{mm}^2)} = 0.127\,\text{mm}$$

For the second implant:

$$\delta = \frac{(1000\,\text{N})(20\,\text{mm})}{(2\,\text{GPa})((\pi)5^2) - ((\pi)2.5^2)} = 0.17\,\text{mm}$$

So both implants move very little when compressed, and the one that experiences more stress has a larger deformation.

This can also be used in cases where multiple forces are placed onto the object or if the object is composed of multiple materials (or a combination of the two). In these cases, the equation becomes:

$$\delta = \sum_i \frac{P_i L_i}{E_i A_i}$$

PROBLEM 1.6

You are evaluating a new device designed to regenerate articular cartilage by replacing the cartilage and a portion of the bone beneath it. The construct will be subjected to a compressive force of 10 N. The diameter of the cartilage portion is 5 mm and the diameter of the bone portion is 7 mm. The modulus of the cartilage and bone sections are 0.75 MPa and 2 GPa, respectively (Figure 1.7).

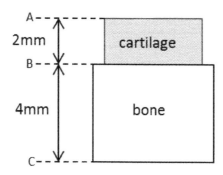

FIGURE 1.7   Schematic of a piece of cartilage on top of bone.

We will solve the problem into the cartilage portion and bone portion.
For the cartilage portion:

$$\delta_c = \frac{PL_c}{E_c A_c} = \frac{(10\,\text{N})(2\,\text{mm})}{(0.75\,\text{MPa})(\pi)(2.5\,\text{mm}^2)} = 1.36\,\text{mm}$$

For the bone portion:

$$\delta_b = \frac{PL_b}{E_b A_b} = \frac{(10\,\text{N})(4\,\text{mm})}{(2\,\text{GPa})(\pi)(3.5\,\text{mm}^2)} = 5.2 \times 10^{-4}\,\text{mm}$$

$$\delta_{\text{total}} = 1.36052\,\text{mm} \approx 1.36\,\text{mm}$$

Just like force can be normalized to form stress, deformation can be normalized to form strain. A tensile stress creates a positive strain, an increase in length, whereas compressive stress creates a negative strain, a decrease in length. If you had a small rubber bar with a length L_0 and stretched it an additional amount ΔL the new length L would be $L + \Delta L$. The stretched ratio, L_0/L, is noted by λ. There are two types of strains, engineering strain and true strain. Engineering strain is calculated with reference to the original length, and true strain is calculated with reference to the length after the strain.

$$\varepsilon = \frac{l - l_0}{l_0} = \frac{\Delta l}{l_0} = \lambda - 1 \qquad \text{Engineering Strain}$$

$$\varepsilon = \frac{l - l_0}{l} = 1 - \frac{1}{\lambda} \qquad \text{True Strain}$$

where l_0 is the original length, l is the length after the strain has taken place, and λ is the strain ratio. Engineering strain will be used throughout this book.

Just as there are different types of stress there are also different types of strain. The strains in equations are examples of normal strain. Normal strain leads to tension, an increase in the length, or compression, a decrease in the length (Figure 1.8).

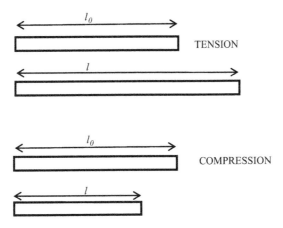

FIGURE 1.8   Examples of strains caused by tension and compression.

PROBLEM 1.7

In Problem 1.5 we observed the behavior of two regenerative bone implants. Using the data from that problem, find the strain in each implant using the same loading conditions. We need to convert the deformation into a strain using Equation 1.4.

For the first implant:

$$\varepsilon = \frac{0.127\,\text{mm}}{20\,\text{mm}} = 6.35 \times 10^{-3} = 0.635\%$$

For the second implant:

$$\varepsilon = \frac{0.17\,\text{mm}}{20\,\text{mm}} = 8.5 \times 10^{-3} = 0.85\%$$

In these equations epsilon is the strain. Note that the strains have been converted into percentages by dividing by 100.

Along with being able to measure the stress experienced by the scaffold that you have produced, you must also be able to mechanically characterize the scaffold to prove that it is appropriate to replace a specific tissue. These properties include elastic modulus, Poisson's ratio, and shear modulus.

The elastic modulus is a measure of material stiffness. If you were to apply an increasing amount of stress to an object and measure the change in the strain as a result of the stress and plot it, the slope of that plot would be the modulus. It is the change in stress divided by the change in strain.

$$E = \frac{\sigma}{\varepsilon} \qquad\qquad \text{Elastic modulus}$$

This relationship is called *Hooke's Law* and can be arranged as:

$$\sigma = E\varepsilon \qquad\qquad \text{Hooke's Law}$$

In these equations, E is the elastic modulus, σ is the stress, and ε is the strain.

As the elastic modulus of a material increases, the material becomes stiffer and more brittle. Bone, for example, is more brittle than cartilage; so bone has a larger elastic modulus than cartilage.

The stress-strain behavior can also be described using stress-strain curve. A stress-strain curve plots the changes in the stress experienced by a material as the material is being strained. The strain could be positive (tension), or negative (compression). As the strain changes, there is a corresponding change in the stress. The two are plotted together to create a stress-strain curve (Figure 1.9).

The straight portion of each plot is the elastic region. This region follows Hooke's Law; therefore their slopes are the elastic moduli of the tested materials. The plastic region follows this, where the relationship between stress and strain changes. The stress represented by point A on each curve is the ultimate stress, the largest value for stress on the curve. Point B is the yield stress, where the behavior of the material begins to change from elastic

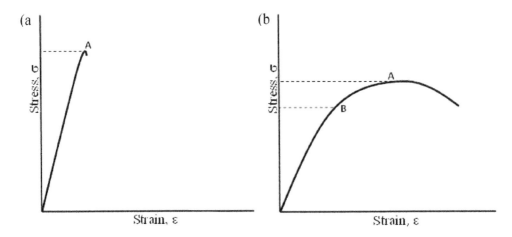

FIGURE 1.9   Stress-strain curves for (a) brittle and (b) ductile materials.

to plastic. In the elastic region, the strain causes no permanent damage to the material; if you release the stress while in this region, the strain returns to zero. In the plastic region, increases in strain lead to more permanent damage to the material; this is *plastic deformation*. If you release the stress while in this region, the strain will not return to zero.

The work done on a material to stretch it within the elastic region is called the *modulus of resiliency*. It is found by calculating the area under the elastic region of the stress strain-curve. All of this energy is recoverable when the applied force is removed. The modulus of toughness is the total energy a material can absorb before fracture and is the area under the entire stress-strain curve. For ductile materials, this is the area under the elastic and plastic regions. The inclusion of fibrous, ductile components to brittle materials can increase the toughness of the composite. This is how bone gains its toughness; bone is a composite of fibrous collagen and a ceramic phase of calcium phosphate.

In Figure 1.9, the first plot is the stress-strain curve for a brittle material, and the second plot is the stress-strain curve for a ductile material. As a brittle material is loaded, there is a large change in stress for a small change in strain. Brittle materials have no yield stress, and rupture occurs without a noticeable change in slope. The breaking stress is the ultimate stress. Ceramics used in bone tissue engineering are examples of brittle materials.

A ductile material has the ability to yield at normal temperature. As the material is loaded, its length increases linearly at a slow rate. After the yield stress is reached, the specimen undergoes large deformations with small increases in stress. This causes a decrease in the slope of the curve and then there is failure. Many of the polymers used in degradable matrices, such as poly ε-caprolactone, are ductile materials.

Some materials display an additional region in their stress-strain curves. The curves display a low slope region that is followed by the linear region (Figure 1.10). Soft biological tissues display this type of behavior. You begin with a region of very low slope and then transition into a high slope region. This low slope area is called the *toe region* and is caused by the straightening and alignment of the collagen fibers that make up the tissue. So in the beginning when the stress is first added to the tissue, that stress is used to alter the geometry of the collagen fibers. Therefore, the fibers are bearing very little load, causing only a small

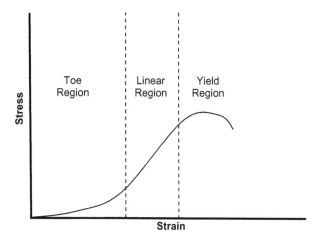

FIGURE 1.10   Stress-strain curve for soft collagenous tissues.

increase in stress as a function of strain. Once they have been straightened and aligned, the collagen fibers now bear *all* of the applied load and the tissue assumes a "normal" stress strain curve. This is the *linear region*. Here the collagen molecules and the crosslinks bear the load. In the yield and failure region, the load is large enough to break the crosslinks and bonds that hold the collagen fibrils together, leading to tissue failure. This is *defibrillation*.

1.5 POISSON'S RATIO

When you pull a material in one direction (creating tension and increasing the length), the material decreases in length in the transverse directions. Although we don't account for it in statics, stresses in one direction have consequences in other directions. This is extremely important when we are talking about load-bearing tissues such as tendons and ligaments. If I am testing a ligament under tension along the y-axis, there will be a decrease in the size in the two transverse directions (x and z). Because the tensile stress in the applied force is divided by the cross-sectional area, I must be able to account for these changes as they affect the cross-sectional area, and therefore, affect my stress measurements.

The relationship between the strain in one direction and the corresponding strain in the transverse direction is called the *Poisson's ratio*. Poisson's ratio is given by the following equation:

$$\nu = -\left|\frac{\text{lateral strain}}{\text{axial strian}}\right| = -\frac{\varepsilon_y}{\varepsilon_x} = -\frac{\varepsilon_z}{\varepsilon_x} \qquad \text{Poisson's ratio}$$

Because this is a relationship between strains, we can insert this into Hooke's Law. Remember, according to Hooke's Law:

$$\varepsilon_x = \frac{\sigma_x}{E}, \text{ therefore } \varepsilon_y = \varepsilon_z = -\frac{\nu\varepsilon_x}{E}$$

This allows us to measure how the application of load in one direction affects strain in another direction. This relationship holds true in the linear region of the stress-strain curve.

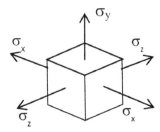

FIGURE 1.11   A cube with normal forces on every face.

The Poisson's ratio is affected by the structure of the scaffold. Are the fibers in the scaffolds randomly oriented or linearly arranged? Is the scaffold dense or very porous? Each of these properties can increase or decrease Poisson's ratio.

Let's say we have a cube that has a normal force on every face (Figure 1.11):

If the original length of each side is 1, the lengths following the application of the stresses are:

$$1+\varepsilon_x, 1+\varepsilon_y, \text{ and } 1+\varepsilon_z$$

Using Hooke's Law, we can relate the strains in each direction in terms of the stresses in each direction using the principle of superposition. This principle states that the effect of combined loading on a structure can be calculated by determining the effects of the different loads separately and then combining them.

$$\varepsilon_x = \frac{\sigma_x}{E} - \frac{v\sigma_y}{E} - \frac{v\sigma_z}{E} \qquad \text{Generalized Hooke's Law}$$

$$\varepsilon_y = \frac{-v\sigma_x}{E} + \frac{\sigma_y}{E} - \frac{v\sigma_z}{E}$$

$$\varepsilon_z = \frac{-v\sigma_x}{E} - \frac{v\sigma_y}{E} + \frac{\sigma_z}{E}$$

These equations are known as the *Generalized Hooke's Law*. For this to work, the following conditions must be true:

- The strain must be below the proportionality limit, in the linear region of the stress-strain curve.

- Each effect is linearly related to the load producing it.

- The deformation from a load is so small that it does not affect the application of the other loads.

The Generalized Hooke's Law gives us a way to quantify how a stress in one direction affects a material in other directions. We can use it for cases when an object is subjected to multiple forces from multiple directions. We can break up the forces into their x, y, and z components, find the corresponding stresses, and plug them into the equations. Based on the strains that we calculate, we can decide it the design for our device is flawed. If the strain is too large, we can change the material used (this alters the modulus, E) or change the dimensions (this alters the area, which alters the stress).

PROBLEM 1.8

A hydrogel for use as a regenerative replacement for cartilage is being tested to evaluate its mechanical behavior. To see how the material behaves when experiencing normal stresses from different directions, you subject it to a uniform pressure, σ, on all sides (Figure 1.12). Assume $E = 72.5$ psi and $v = 0.3$. You have observed that the change in length of edge AB is -1.2×10^{-3} inches, calculate the change in length of the other two edges, CB and BD (12 points) and the pressure, σ, applied to the faces of the sample.

We will use our Generalized Hooke's Law equations, but first we must convert the change in length into a strain.

$$\Delta AB = -1.2 \times 10^{-3} \text{ in} \therefore \varepsilon_x = \frac{-1.2 \times 10^{-3} \text{ in}}{4 \text{ in}} = -3 \times 10^{-4}$$

Now use the Generalized Hooke's Law

$$\varepsilon_x = \frac{\sigma_x}{E} - v\frac{\sigma_y}{E} - v\frac{\sigma_z}{E} = \frac{1}{E}(\sigma - v(\sigma + \sigma)) = \frac{1}{E}(\sigma - 2v\sigma) = \frac{\sigma}{E}(1 - 2v)$$

$$\therefore \sigma = \frac{\varepsilon_x E}{(1 - 2v)}$$

Now we can plug in our known variables to find the stress

$$\sigma = \frac{(-3 \times 10^{-4}) \times (72.5)}{(1 - 0.6)} = 5.4 \times 10^{-2} \text{ psi}$$

Now that we know the stress, we can find the strains and convert them into changes in length

$$\varepsilon_y = \frac{\sigma}{E}(1 - 2v) = -3 \times 10^{-4} \left(\text{same as } \varepsilon_x\right)$$

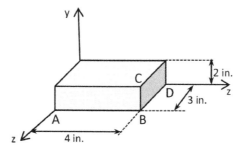

FIGURE 1.12   A hydrogel subjected to uniform pressure.

$$\Delta CB = \varepsilon_y \times \overline{CB} = (-3\times10^{-4})(2\,\text{in}) = -6\times10^{-4}\,\text{in}$$

$$\Delta DB = \varepsilon_z \times \overline{DB} = (-3\times10^{-4})(3\,\text{in}) = -9\times10^{-4}\,\text{in}$$

1.6 SHEAR STRESSES, TORSION, AND BENDING

In the previous sections, we examined the concept of stress. In particular we discussed normal stresses that lead to tension and compression and their corresponding strains (changes in length). We will continue the discussion of stress, but we will look into the effects of stresses that are acting directly down the primary axis of an object. Specifically, we will discuss shear stresses and stresses that lead to torsion and bending. These concepts are important because tissues experience a variety of stresses from a variety of directions; so tissue-engineered devices must be able to withstand stresses that create shear, bending, and twisting.

1.7 SHEAR STRESS

Up to this point, we have been discussing normal stresses, stresses that are applied to an object 90° to its surface. Obviously this is not the only type of loading situation that exists. Along with forces that are applied normal to a surface, we can also have forces that are applied parallel to the surface. Shearing stresses occur when a force acts parallel to a surface or two transverse forces are applied to a member. In both cases the forces are acting along a plane (parallel to it) creating a shear stress along the plane. The magnitude of a shear stress can be found using the following equation:

$$\tau = \frac{P}{A}$$

where τ is the shear stress, P is the force and A is the area of the surface that the force is acting on. This equation is very similar to the equation for normal stress; the difference lies in the direction of P. In the previous equation, P is acting perpendicular to the surface; in this equation, P is acting parallel to the surface. This is actually an average shear stress; the true shearing stress is not assumed to be uniform. The application of a shear stress yields a shear strain; this is an *angular deformation* (Figure 1.13).

Shear stress can also be experienced by a material internally. A normal force can cause shearing stresses on adjacent planes, or two forces of equal magnitude but opposite direction can cause a shearing stress when they are separated by a plane (Figure 1.14).

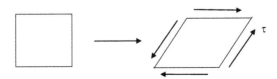

FIGURE 1.13   A change in shape as a result of shear strain caused by shear stress.

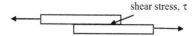

shear stress, τ

FIGURE 1.14 Shear stress as a result of two forces of equal magnitude but opposite direction separated by a plane.

Shearing stresses are common in biomedical engineering. Along with compression, articular cartilage experiences a great deal of shear. When joints bend, the cartilage at the ends of the bones rotate along each other. By simply washing your face, you are placing a shearing stress on your skin. In tissue engineering, a smooth lubricated surface must be created for any potentially implantable cartilage scaffold. Internal shear can also be experienced within tissues when they experience multiple loads from opposing directions or loads that cause twisting (this will be discussed later).

Fluid flow over a surface is another source of shear, a major example of this is seen in blood vessels. Along with being able to withstand pulsatile forces crated by the pumping of blood through the circulatory systems, the inside of any potential scaffolding for vascular regeneration must be able to withstand the constant shear stresses exerted by blood flow without wearing down or tearing the inner surface. A simplistic look at this kind of shear stress is given using the following equation for flow of a liquid between two plates:

$$\tau = \mu \frac{dv}{dy}$$

Here τ is the shear stress, μ is the viscosity of the liquid, and dv/dy notes the change in fluid velocity as a function of your position vertically between the plates. According to this equation, an increase in the viscosity of the solution increases the shear stress exerted by the fluid onto the walls. The shear stress exerted onto the walls by the fluid also increases with an increase in fluid velocity (dv increases) or the closer you are to the walls (dy decreases), as seen in Figure 1.2. This equation assumes that the fluid flow is laminar.

1.7.1 Shearing Strain

Shearing stresses have no direct effect on the normal strains. They will tend to deform a cube into an oblique parallelepiped (Figure 1.15). The change in the angle between sides A and B is the shear strain, γ. Therefore, we can redraw the previous figure as (Figure 1.16):

γ_{xy} = change in angle = shearing strain

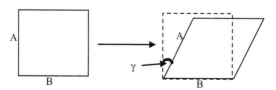

FIGURE 1.15 Shearing strains deform a cube into an oblique parallelepiped.

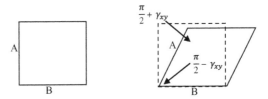

FIGURE 1.16 Shearing strains caused by a shearing force.

You can plot τ_{xy} vs γ_{xy} for a shearing stress-strain diagram and obtain the following relation:

$$\tau_{xy} = G(\gamma_{xy}) \qquad\qquad \text{Hooke's Law for shear}$$

The same holds true for the shear stresses in the other directions

$$\tau_{yz} = G(\gamma_{yz}) \qquad \tau_{zx} = G(\gamma_{zx})$$

where G is the shear modulus or modulus of rigidity. In general, the value of G is between 0.33 E and 0.5 E, where E is the elastic modulus.

PROBLEM 1.9
You are testing a potential skin substitute. It is comparable to natural skin in tension, but it has not been examined under shear. You have bonded a piece of the skin substitute (50 mm long, 50 mm wide, 2 mm thick) to the base of the machine and subjected the top surface to a shear force. The shear strain is monitored by a camera. You apply a force of 100 N to the entire surface of the material and observe a shear strain of $\pi/5$. What are shear stress experienced by the material and the shear modulus of the material?

A force on 100 N is placed over the sample, which has a surface area of 250 mm. Therefore,

$$\frac{100 \text{ N}}{250 \text{ mm}} = 0.4 \text{ MPa}$$

With a measured shear strain of $\pi/5$ the shear modulus is

$$\frac{0.4 \text{ MPa}}{\pi/5} = 0.022 \text{ MPa}$$

1.7.2 Internal Shear and Relating Shear and Normal Stresses

We have described shear stresses and strains in situations where there is a force placing a shear stress on the surface of an object, but shear stresses can also form inside of an object. There are several types of loading conditions that create internal shear, which can lead to failure of a structure (Figure 1.17).

First, let's prove the presence of internal shear with a simple experiment. Previously, when discussing Poisson's ratio and Generalized Hooke's Law, we observed that when a cube with sides of length 1 is subjected to a uniaxial strain the lengths become

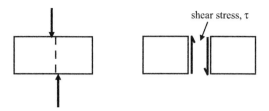

FIGURE 1.17   Diagram of internal shear stress.

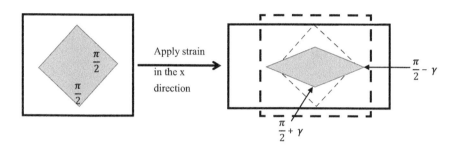

FIGURE 1.18   Converting axial strain into shear strain.

$1 + x$, $1 - x$, $1 - x$. Now let's take a side of that cube and place a smaller square inside of it and rotate it as seen in the Figure 1.18.

If we apply the same strain in the x direction, we can see that although the white outer square elongates into a rectangle (leaving the right angles at the corners intact), the grey inner square becomes a rhombus (changing the angles at the corners). The dashed shapes are the squares before the addition of strain. Because the angles changes from $\pi/4$ to β, we know that there is a shear strain present. This serves as further proof that shearing stresses can develop from axial loading. To relate shear strain to axial loading mathematically, we can solve for β. Because the first angle is half of the original angle, the shearing strain as a result of the axial load will also be half of what it was in the cube. So:

$$\beta = \frac{\pi}{4} - \frac{\gamma_m}{2}$$

Now that we have the length of the sides and a value for the angle, we can create a relationship between the strain from the sides and shear strain from the corner. First we use the formula for the tangent of the difference of two angles. This gives us:

$$\tan\beta = \frac{\tan\dfrac{\pi}{4} - \tan\dfrac{\gamma_m}{2}}{1 + \tan\dfrac{\pi}{4}\tan\dfrac{\gamma_m}{2}} = \frac{1 - \tan\dfrac{\gamma_m}{2}}{1 + \tan\dfrac{\gamma_m}{2}}$$

We will assume that γ_m is very small, so:

$$\tan\beta = \frac{1 - \dfrac{\gamma_m}{2}}{1 + \dfrac{\gamma_m}{2}}$$

Using the lengths of the sides, we can write:

$$\tan\beta = \frac{1 - \nu\varepsilon_x}{1 + \varepsilon_x}$$

$$\therefore \tan\beta = \frac{1 - \nu\varepsilon_x}{1 + \varepsilon_x} = \frac{1 - \dfrac{\gamma_m}{2}}{1 + \dfrac{\gamma_m}{2}}$$

and

$$\gamma_m = \frac{(1 + \nu)\varepsilon_x}{1 + \dfrac{1 - \nu}{2}\varepsilon_x}$$

Since ε_x is much smaller than 1, the denominator can be assumed to be equal to 1. So:

$$\gamma_m = (1 + \nu)\varepsilon_x$$

This gives us a relation between γ_m and ε_x, shearing strain and axial strain.

In addition, there is a relationship between the elastic modulus and shear modulus.

$$\frac{E}{2G} = 1 + \nu \qquad \text{or} \qquad G = \frac{E}{2(1 + \nu)}$$

Why are all of these concepts important? Shear stress is experienced by many tissues in the body. In particular internal shear is extremely important when it comes to failure analysis. By measuring the shear stresses placed on a scaffold or experienced within the scaffolds you can discover if the scaffold will fail once it is implanted and experiences the forces placed on it by the body.

PROBLEM 1.10

You are designing a scaffold for ligament replacement. Although most people think of ligament as a tissue that is subjected to tensile stresses, you realize that these tensile forces can lead to the creation of shear strains. Therefore, you want to examine your tensile data and use it to estimate the maximum shear strain of the scaffold. The material has an elastic modulus, E, of 300 MPa, Poisson's ratio of 0.4, and an ultimate tensile stress of 100 MPa.

We are going to make an assumption that your material is linearly elastic, so we can use Hooke's Law to help us solve for the shear strain. So according to Hooke's Law:

$$\sigma = E\varepsilon$$

Plugging in our values at failure we get

$$100\ \text{MPa} = 300\ \text{MPa} \times \varepsilon \therefore \varepsilon \approx 0.33$$

Now we have a tensile strain to plug into our shear strain equation

$$\gamma_m = (1+v)\varepsilon_x \text{ so } \gamma_m = (1+0.4)0.33 = 0.462$$

So at failure, the scaffold experiences internal shear strains as large as 0.462.

1.8 STRESSES IN BENDING

Previously we examined moments (force × distance) and learned about using moment balances to solve for forces that could be placed on our scaffolds and devices. When two moments of equal magnitude and opposite direction combine as shown in Figure 1.19, bending occurs.

In this figure, A B is a beam under a constant bending moment. You may ask why is this important for tissue engineering. We don't bend during normal, everyday activities. In actuality, we do bend, the magnitude of the bending is very small. The most-often studied cases of bending are in orthopedics. Load-bearing bones are placed under forces that can lead to bending during everyday activities. Walking, running, lifting, and carrying items can create moments that lead to slight amounts of bending in bone. As biomedical engineers building bone replacements or regenerating bone, we need to be certain that our scaffolds or newly regenerated tissues can withstand these moments without bending more than normal bone.

Two things happen when an object is bent. One side increases in length (placed under tension) and the other side decreases in length (placed under compression; Figure 1.20). If this were a cell-seeded scaffold, this tension or compression would be felt by the cells in the

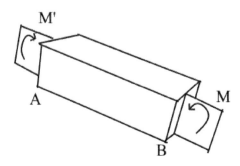

FIGURE 1.19 Diagram of a beam under a pair of moments that are equal in magnitude and opposite in direction.

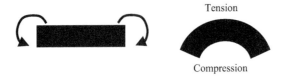

Tension

Compression

FIGURE 1.20 Pure bending produces both tension and compression in the same object.

scaffold. So it is important to learn how to calculate the tensile and compressive stresses and strains caused be bending. We will take rectangular beam and place it under moments M and M'. To find the stresses in the beam, we must first find the deformations and strains.

So what happens when we bend an object with equal and opposite couples M and M'? In Figure 1.21, the points A and B and A' and B' remain in the same plane. The line AB or A'B' becomes part of a circle with center C (lines AB and A'B' have a constant curvature). The length of AB↓ is less than the length of A'B'↑, so the top is in compression and bottom in tension. Therefore, there must be a surface or plane perpendicular to both AB and A'B'; where we switch from tension (which has a positive sign) to compression (which has a negative sign). So at this surface or plane, the strain and stress would equal zero. This is the neutral surface or neutral axis (Figure 1.21). In a rectangular beam, the neutral axis lies in the middle of the beam (from the top) because of symmetry. If it were a prism, the neutral axis would be closer to the wider end.

The strains and their corresponding stresses vary linearly throughout the thickness of the beam from compression at the top to tension at the bottom. In this case, the strain reaches its most positive value (largest tensile strain) at the very bottom and its most negative value (largest compressive strain) at the very top. Because in a linearly elastic material, strain is proportional to stress, the stress also changes in the same way.

So how do we calculate the strain? We start by calculating the deformation, how much it moves as a result of bending. Once again we'll take the origin at the neutral axis. We will relate the deformation based on the arc described previously (Figure 1.22).

Looking at the diagram of the beam undergoing bending, we can see that the original length of the beam, L, is the length of the neutral surface which is

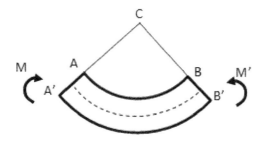

FIGURE 1.21 A beam bent under 2 moments. The dashed line represents the neutral axis, the place where the normal stress is zero.

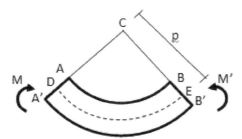

FIGURE 1.22   A more in-depth look at a beam bent under 2 moments. The length of DE = Length of undeformed member L. The radius = p (at arc DE). Θ = central angle.

$$L = p\Theta$$

This length will changes if we go above or below the neutral surface for example: Arc JK is y above neutral surface its length L'

$$L' = (p - y)\Theta$$

Because JK before bending = L

$$\delta = L' - L$$

$$\delta = (p - y)\Theta - p\Theta = -y\Theta$$

Remember that the strain represents the change in length; engineering strain is essentially the percentage of change. So in this case, the strain is:

$$\varepsilon_y = \frac{\delta}{L} = \frac{-y\theta}{p\theta} = \frac{-y}{p}$$

Note that there is a negative y because of a negative bending moment

So according to this equation, ε_y (longitudinal strain) varies linearly with distance y from neutral surface. So the strain reaches its maximum value at the farthest distance from the neutral axis (one of the object faces). Therefore:

$$\varepsilon_{max} = \frac{c}{p} \text{ and } \varepsilon = \frac{-y}{c}\varepsilon_{max}$$

In this equation, c is the maximum distance away from the neutral axis.

So if you know the maximum strain and the dimensions of the object, you can calculate the strain at anywhere throughout the thickness of the object. The strain is also maximum at the top of our object in this example. So if this was a cell-seeded scaffold, the cells that are placed at the top of this scaffold will experience the most strain after bending. There would also be a difference in the strain experienced by the cells as you travel from the top of the scaffold toward the bottom. This is extremely important for cell culture because you may experience differences in cellular behavior based on the differences in strain.

Now let's consider the stress that results from bending in the elastic range.

$$\sigma_x = E\varepsilon_x$$

Substitute from earlier:

$$\sum \varepsilon_x = \left(\frac{-y}{c} \right)$$

$$\sigma_x = \frac{-y}{c} \left(\sigma_{max} \right)$$

σ_x is the normal stress, which varies linearly, and σ_{max} is the maximum absolute value for stress.

Now we will define a simpler equation that we can use to solve for the stress at any plane in an object. We will start by saying that if we bend a symmetric object, we will have equal amounts of compression and tension, so that all of the stress in the object cancel. We can say this using the following equation:

$$\int \sigma_x dA = 0$$

This can be rewritten using our previous equation that links σ_x to σ_{max}, so that:

$$\int \frac{-y}{c} \sigma_{max} dA = 0 = \frac{-\sigma_{max}}{c} A = \int y dA = 0$$

So the first moment of the cross-section about the neutral axis = 0. For this to be true, the stresses must be in elastic range and the neutral axis must pass through centroid (only for pure bending).

Stress is defined as a force divided by the area that it was acting on, and a moment, M, as a force multiplied by the distance that it was acting on. So we can take these two definitions and turn the previous equation into a moment by inserting σ_x, so that:

$$\int -y\sigma_x dA = M$$

Substitute for σ_x

$$\int -y\left(\frac{-y}{c} \right) \sigma_{max} dA = M$$

We can rearrange this to solve for the Moment of Inertia (I) through the centroid:

$$\frac{-\sigma_{max}}{c} \int y^2 dA = M, \text{ where } \int y^2 dA = I$$

TABLE 1.1   Moments of Inertia for Several Shapes

Rectangle		$I = bh^3/12$ $J = bh(b^2 + h^2)/12$	Half of a thin-walled tube	$I_x = 0.095\pi r^3 t$ $I_y = 0.5\pi r^3 t$
Circle		$I = \pi r^4/4$ $J = \pi r^4/2$	Isosceles triangle	$I_x = bh^3/36$ $I_y = hb^3/48$ $J = (4h^2 + 3b^2)bh/144$
Semicircle		$I_x = 0.110\,r^2$ $I_y = r^4/8$	Right triangle	$I_x = bh^3/36$ $I_y = hb^3/48$ $J = (4h^2 + 3b^2)bh/144$
Thin-walled tube		$I = \pi r^3 t$ $J = 2\pi r^3 t$	Ellipse	$I = \pi ab^3/4$ $J = \pi ab(a^2 + b^2)/4$

Note: b = base, h = height, t = thickness, r = radius.

The Moment of Inertia is the resistance of an object to rotation.

So if you let $y = c$, $\sigma_{max} = Mc/I$

For any distance y, $\sigma_y = -My/I$, the negative sign comes from $\sigma_x = -y/c(\sigma_{max})$
In this equation:
Stress is compressive $\sigma_x < 0$ and $y > 0$ above neutral axis M = position
Stress is tensile $\sigma < 0$ and M is negative
The moments of inertia have been defined for many common shapes. They are listed in Table 1.1.

We can further simplify this equation by defining the elastic section modulus, S:

$$S = I/c \text{ therefore } \sigma_m = M/S$$

By definition, S depends on the geometry of your object, so if you want to reduce the amount of stress felt by the object, and lower the chances of it failing, you can alter the geometry so that you reduce the value of S.

PROBLEM 1.11

You are designing a thin, rectangular, plate-like scaffold to regenerate a long bone defect following the removal of a tumor. You have two designs for the scaffold. They both have the same cross-sectional area, but one has a height of 3 mm and the other has a height of 5 mm. The surgeon will shape the defect to match the dimensions of the scaffold. Which design should the surgeon use to minimize the chances of the scaffold breaking once it is implanted?

The design that has less stress placed on it will have a smaller chance of failing, so we must figure out which of the two designs has the lowest value for σ_{max}. We just found that

$\sigma_m = M/S$ and $S = I/c$. If we look at Table 1.1 we can find the equation for the Moment of Inertia, I, for a rectangle. Plugging it into the equation for S we get:

$$S = \frac{I}{c} = \frac{1}{12} \frac{bh^3}{b/2} = \frac{1}{6} Ah$$

In this equation, b is the base, h is the height, and A is the cross-sectional area. So if the two designs have the same value for A, the one with the height of 5 mm will have a larger value of S than the one with a height of 3 mm. Because $\sigma_m = M/S$, the design with the height of 5 mm will experience less stress and therefore have a lower risk of failure.

1.8.1 Bending of a Cantilever Beam

A common problem in mechanical engineering is the bending of a cantilever beam. A cantilever beam is a beam that is attached to an object such as a wall at one end and is free at the other end. In Figure 1.23, the black cantilever beam is attached to the wall (white). If enough force (F) is placed on the beam it will begin to bend.

If the force is placed at the very end of the beam, the distance that the beam moves down in the y direction, the deflection is given by the following equation:

$$y = \frac{F}{EI}\left(\frac{x^3}{6} - \frac{Lx^2}{2}\right)$$

In this equation, F is the applied force, E is the modulus (or stiffness) of the beam, y is the deflection, x is the place on the beam (in the x direction) where you are measuring the deflection, and L is the total beam length. In the case seen in the figure, the maximum deflection is at the end of the beam, so we can calculate the maximum deflection by substituting in L for x. This gives us:

$$y_{max} = \frac{FL^3}{2EI}$$

If a force was placed onto your scaffold, you could measure the amount that it bends with these equations.

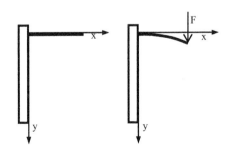

FIGURE 1.23   A cantilever beam bending under a force, F.

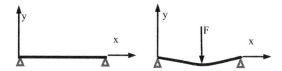

FIGURE 1.24 A supported beam bending as a result of a force placed on the middle of the beam.

Another common type of bending is three-point bending. In this case, a beam is supported at the two ends and a force is placed in the middle (Figure 1.24).

The equations that govern the deflection are:

$$y = \frac{1}{EI}\left(\frac{Fx^3}{12} - \frac{FL^2}{16}x\right) \quad y_{max} = \frac{FL^3}{48EI}$$

This type of test is commonly used for bone tissue. Long bones are subjected to multiple forces that can lead to slight bending. This test allows the engineer to see idf the implant can withstand those forces.

1.9 STRESSES IN TORSION

Another application of moments is torsion. Torsion is another type of loading that occurs in materials including tissues in the body. It is the twisting of an object because of the presence of oppositely directed moments of the same magnitude that produce rotation about the longitudinal axis of that object. These moments are frequently referred to as *twisting couples* or *torques*. In Figure 1.25, they are labeled T and T'.

In biomechanics, torsion occurs in bone. Torsional breaks occur in bone; these breaks occur during skiing when the ski hits object, and the body turns one way and the foot turns the other way. One common test for regenerative bone scaffolds for tissue engineering is the torsional test.

We can define torque by looking at the forces that create torsion. Let's place a torque, T, on a femur and break it into the forces that cause it. Let's look at a section of the femur in Figure 1.26.

So the torque can be converted into moments composed of small forces, dF, that are a perpendicular distance, P, away from the axis. This is represented mathematically by:

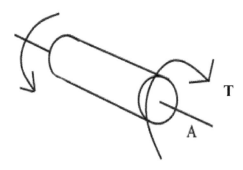

FIGURE 1.25 A rod under torsion because of torques placed at the ends.

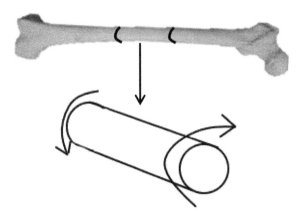

FIGURE 1.26 A closer look at a bone under torsion.

$$\int p\,dF = T$$

This equation gives us the moments of the forces causing torsion. These forces are shearing forces. By definition:

$$\tau = \frac{F}{A}$$

Now substitute it into the torque equation:

$$\therefore dF = \tau\,dA$$

So now the torque equation becomes:

$$\int p(\tau\,dA) = T$$

We have looked at the stresses that cause torsion, what kind of deformation results from torsion?

We will begin with a cylinder bound at one end and apply a torque, T, to free end. What happens to the shape of a rectangular section of the cylinder after torsion?

When we apply the torsion, the position of the left and right sides remain the same, but the top and bottom are tilted and the corner angles have changed (Figure 1.27). This is proof of the presence of shear stress and shear strain (as defined in the previous section). For small values of γ, arc length $AA' = L\gamma$. We also know that $AA' = p\Phi$, so by substitution, $L\gamma = p\Phi$. Therefore:

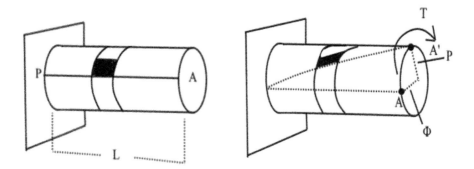

FIGURE 1.27   Distortion of a rectangle drawn on a rod after torsion is applied. The change in the angles is proof of the presence of shear strain.

$$\gamma = \frac{\rho\Phi}{L}$$

According to this equation, the shear strain, γ, varies linearly with the distance away from axis of the shaft, p, so shear stress is max on the surface where $p = c$, where c is the maximum distance from the center, this is similar to what we saw in bending. So therefore:

$$\gamma_{max} = \frac{c\Phi}{L} \quad \text{and} \quad \gamma = \frac{\rho}{c}\gamma_{max}$$

Just like normal stress being related to strain through Hooke's Law and the use of the elastic modulus, E, shear stress and shear strain are also related through Hooke's Law for shear stress and the shear modulus, G.

$$\tau = G\gamma$$

So because γ varies with the distance from the center, according to Hooke's Law the same relationship should exist for the shear stress, τ.
    So:

$$\gamma = \frac{\rho}{c}\gamma_{max}$$

This can be represented by Figure 1.28.
    The minimum stress, τ_{min}, is zero and occurs at the center. If the cylinder is hollow as seen in bone, τ_{min} is not zero and does not occur at the center (Figure 1.28).

$$\frac{\tau_{min}}{c_1} = \frac{\tau_{max}}{c_2} \quad \text{and} \quad \tau_{min} = \frac{c_1}{c_2}\tau_{max}$$

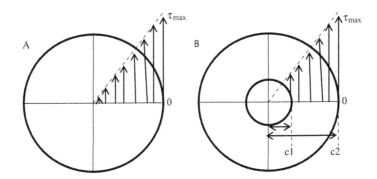

FIGURE 1.28   Shear stress profile in the cross-section of rods under torsion. Rod A is solid; Rod B is hollow.

Now we want to relate torque placed onto the cylinder with the shear stress created in the cylinder. Let's begin with our previous equation for torque.

$$\int p(\tau dA) = T$$

Now substitute in the equation for maximum shear stress:

$$\int p(\tau dA) = T = \frac{\tau_{max}}{c} \int p^2 dA$$

By definition:

$$\int p^2 dA = J, \text{ the polar moment of inertia}$$

For a cylinder of radius c:

$$J = \frac{\pi c^4}{2}$$

For a hollow cylinder:

$$J = \frac{\pi \left(c_2^4 - c_1^4 \right)}{2}$$

$$T = \frac{\tau_{max} J}{c} \therefore \tau_{max} = \frac{Tc}{J} \text{ and } \tau = \frac{Tp}{J}$$

Where p is any distance away from the center.

As we saw in this section, tensile stresses can lead to shear stresses; the converse is also true: shear stress can create tensile stress. If we look at an element in a cylinder under

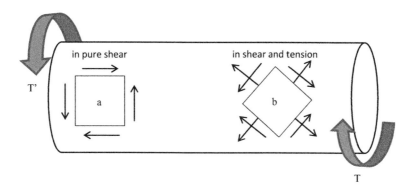

FIGURE 1.29 The relationship between the orientation of an element and the forces that it experiences. The straight square on the left is under pure shear, whereas the square on the right experiences shear and tension.

torsion we can see that the forces on the element change as the orientation of the element changes (Figure 1.29). In Figure 1.29, the element on the left experiences only shear forces; therefore, the stress is the maximum shear force. The element on the right experiences a mixture of forces. As you can see, the forces placed on the element change when the orientation of the element is changed. To figure out why let's take a look inside of the element on the left. Specifically, we will take a 45° cut into the element from the cylinder axis (Figure 1.30).

Because the stresses on BC and BD equal to τ_{max} (remember $\tau_{max} = Tc/J$), so their forces are equal to the stress multiplied by the area upon which they are applied, A_0. The force F is perpendicular to the faces DC anc BE. Through geometry we find that:

$$F = 2\left(\tau_{max} A_0\right)\cos 45° = \tau_{max} A_0 \sqrt{2}$$

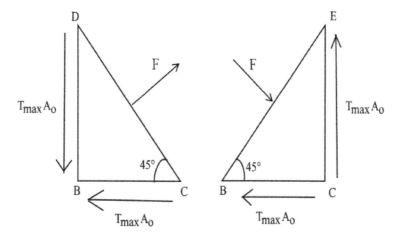

FIGURE 1.30 A look at the forces inside of a small element in a rod experiencing tension. We can see that the type of force and its magnitude depend on the angle of the surface experiencing the force.

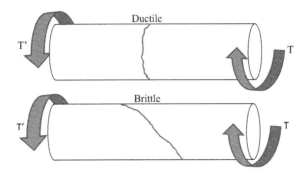

FIGURE 1.31   Modes of failure for ductile materials and brittle materials when placed under torsion.

Remember, this is a force to get a stress. Divide by area:

$$\tau_{max} \frac{A_0\sqrt{2}}{A_0\sqrt{2}} = \tau_{max}$$

So on DC:

$$\sigma = \tau_{max}$$

and BE:

$$\sigma = -\tau_{max}$$

Now this is interesting, but why is it practical? If we know the mechanical properties of our device, we can Figure out how they will behave and fail under torsion. For example, when we place a device under torsion, we can get forces that look like those seen in Figure 1.29. So let's say that our material is ductile. In general, ductile materials are weakest under shear. According to Figure 1.29, the highest level of shear stress is transverse to the device long axis. Therefore we would expect the device to fail along this plane (Figure 1.31).

Here is another example: You are now testing a brittle bone replacement device under torsion. Analyses have shown that brittle materials are weakest under tension. According to our prior analysis, the tensile stress placed on the device when it is under torsion is equal to the maximum shear stress at an angle 45° off of the long axis. So you would expect for it to break in this direction (Figure 1.31). This actually happens in real life; it is called a *spiral fracture* and is seen when bones are placed under torsion (Figure 1.32).

1.9.1 Torsional Shear Strain

In torsion, we measure strain by observing how much the object has been twisted. This is done by measuring the angle of twist, ϕ, as a result of the torque, T. These calculations will only work if Hooke's Law is accurate; so our stress and strain lie on the straight portion of the stress-strain curve.

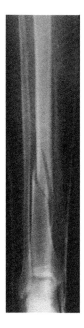

FIGURE 1.32 This X-ray image displays a spiral fracture in a tibia. These breaks occur in cases when the body is in motion while the limb (in this case the leg) is planted. This creates torsion at the limb, which leads to the fracture.

Remember that

$$\gamma_{max} = \frac{c\Phi}{L} \quad \text{and} \quad \gamma = \frac{\rho}{c}\gamma_{max}$$

Since

$$\tau = G\gamma$$

$$\tau_{max} = G\gamma_{max} \text{ so } \gamma_{max} = \frac{\tau_{max}}{G}$$

Substituting in $\tau_{max} = \dfrac{Tc}{J}$

$$\gamma_{max} = \frac{TC}{JG} = \frac{c\phi}{L}$$

After rearranging the equation

$$\phi = \frac{LT}{GJ} \quad \text{where } \phi \text{ is in radians}$$

We can use this equation to calculate how much rotation will occur because of an applied torque, or if you apply a torque and induce the rotation in your scaffold, you can use the equation to solve for the shear modulus, G. Using a torsion testing machine, you can test a sample of length, L, by applying a torque, T. You can then take the slope of your plot (JG/L), calculate J (the polar moment of inertia) and solve for G.

The polar moment of inertia measures the resistance of an object to torsion and is found using the equation:

$$J_0 = \int_A p^2 \, dA$$

Where A is the area, and p is the distance to the point where you are taking the measurement. The values for the polar moments of inertia (J) for common shapes are listed in Table 1.1.

1.10 IMPORTANCE TO TISSUE ENGINEERING

At a first glance, many of these concepts may not seem important for tissue engineers. There is no information about cells or growth factors (this is seen later in the book). Although cells and growth factors, whether exogenous or produced by the cells, are essential to tissue engineering, the application of force, stresses felt by cells, and the elastic modulus of the materials that cells lie on have an important effect on cellular behavior. Cells alter their behavior in response to applied force or stress. Numerous studies have shown that cellular proliferation, differentiation, or extracellular matrix development can be enhanced with the application of stress. On the other hand, too much stress can pull cells from a substrate or cause them to change their shape from extended to spherical. The application of too much stress can cause cell death.

The modulus, or stiffness, of the cellular substrate is also extremely important. The stiffness of the substrate also affects cellular behavior and differentiation. Different cell types prefer different degrees of stiffness. Osteoblasts prefer high modulus materials; fibroblasts prefer less stiff, more flexible materials. Researchers in stem cell biology have shown that their differentiation can be controlled by substrate stiffness. Stem cells have been differentiated into osteoblasts, chondrocytes, and other cell types by controlling the stiffness of the hydrogel that they were seeded on.

In addition, all of these concepts are important if we wish to implant our devices. As stated, our bodies are constantly moving. They are generating forces or being subjected to forces. Therefore, if something is going to be implanted into the body, it must be able to withstand these forces without permanently deforming or breaking. Learning how to analyze stresses and strains will allow a tissue engineer to know how his or her device will perform when implanted and decide if it will thrive in the body or fail. If the analysis points to failure, the concepts in this chapter will allow the engineer to alter the design to better survive the dynamic environment of the human body.

QUESTIONS

1. Another actor is rehearsing for the new *Conan* movie. He is using a sword that weighs 6 N. He holds the sword upright at the center of mass of his hands. What is external

torque on the glenohumeral joint (force on the deltoid tendon)? What are the reaction forces at the shoulder (Rx and Ry)? Remember the deltoid tendon forms an angle of 15° with the humerus and attaches at a point on the humerus 0.12 m away from the shoulder. The other lengths are:

0.59 m from shoulder to the force from the hand.

0.36 m from shoulder to the force from the forearm.

0.13 m from shoulder to the force from the upper arm.

2. You are testing a material for a bone scaffold. A rod of the material is 15 cm long and must not stretch more than 1.2 mm when a 8.5-kN load is applied to it. Knowing that $E = 800$ MPa, determine (a) the smallest diameter rod that should be used, (b) the corresponding normal stress caused by the load.

3. A material used in a scaffold is subjected to a biaxial loading that results in normal stresses $\sigma_x = 120$ MPa and $\sigma_z = 160$ MPa. Knowing that the properties of the polymer can be approximated as $E = 8.7$ GPa and $v = 0.34$, determine the strain in side AB and side BC.

4. You have been given a sample of ligament tissue for mechanical testing. Knowing that the stress at the end of the toe region is 1 MPA, and the modulus of the tissue (for the linear region) is 400 MPa, estimate the stress at a strain of 15% after the toe region.

5. A piece of older skin is subjected to a biaxial load that results in a normal stresses $\sigma_x = 12$ MPa and $\sigma_z = 16$ MPa. Knowing that the average modulus (E) is 0.8 MPa, the Poisson's ratio is 0.34, and the toe length is 0.3 with an increase in stress of 1000 Pa, determine the change in length of

a. side AB

b. side BC

c. diagonal AC

Assume that the material is linearly elastic (all of our simplistic equations apply) after the toe region.

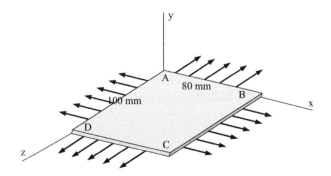

6. You have been hired to design a new ski boot that prevents injuries caused by twisting of the lower leg when the ski hits an object at an angle. Knowing that the average dimensions of the human tibia and the average shear stress of the bone, what is the minimum amount of torque that your boot should be designed for?

Outer diameter = 76 mm

Inner diameter = 9.52

$$\tau_{max} = 60 \text{ MPa}$$

$$J = \pi/2 \, (c^4)$$

c = the overall radius

Hint: Solve for the J of the inner and outer cylinder and subtract the inner from the outer.

7. You are leading a group that is testing a hollow composite rod under torsion. The rod is 20 cm long with an inner diameter of 2 cm and outer diameter of 3 cm. It is composed of a material that has a shear modulus, G, of 0.4 MPa. After looking at the data, you realize that the group forgot to record the magnitude of the torque that they applied. With the given information and knowing that the rod was twisted 2.5 degrees, how much torque was applied to the end of the rod?

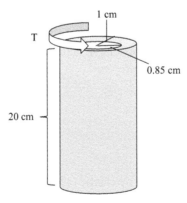

8. There is another version of this scaffold that you have designed has two layers. The outer layer is made up of a polymer-ceramic composite (G = 80 MPa), and the core is completely ceramic (G = 150 MPa). Based on the dimensions supplied in the figure, if the maximum allowable stress is 150 MPa in the ceramic core and 85 MPa in the composite layer, what is the maximum allowable torque that can be placed at the end of the device?

REFERENCES

1. Beer FP, Johnston ER et al. *Mechanics of Materials*. 3rd ed. Europe: McGraw-Hill; 2001.
2. Meriam JL, Kraige LG. *Engineering Mechanics: Statics*. 4th ed. New York: Wiley; 1996.
3. Denard PJ, Dai X et al. Anatomy of the biceps tendon: implications for restoring physiological length-tension relation during biceps tenodesis with interference screw fixation. *Arthroscopy*. 2012 28(10):1352–1358.
4. Stadnick ME. Pathology of the long head of the biceps tendon: Radsource; 2014. Available from: http://radsource.us/pathology-of-the-long-head-of-the-biceps-tendon/.

CHAPTER 2

Heat Transfer and Diffusion

2.1 INTRODUCTION

Along with resisting physical stresses that can lead to cell damage and acting as a physical support for cells, tissues must support the viability of the cells that they house in other ways. Cells need an environment that is physically stable, has the correct temperature, and allows for the flow of nutrients and removal of waste products. When choosing media for cell culture, materials for scaffold construction, and designs for tissue-engineered devices, we cannot just focus on the mechanical properties of the replacement or nutritional supplements for cellular development. We must also consider the ability of the device and culture media to transfer heat to and from the cells and the effect of the media and device porosity to move nutrients to, and waste products from, the cells. Therefore, heat transfer and diffusion play major roles in the survival of cells in a matrix and function of a tissue *in vivo*. As in other areas of this book, this chapter is only providing an introduction to heat transfer in diffusion. For a more in-depth analysis, the reader is referred to texts that focus on these subjects such as *Analysis of Transport Phenomena* by William Deen or *Fundamentals of Momentum, Heat, and Mass Transfer* by James Welty, Charles Wicks, Robert Wilson, and Gregory Rorrer.[1,2] Both of these texts were used as resources for this chapter.

2.2 HEAT TRANSFER

The ability to store, generate, and dispose of heat is extremely important to human life. The human body strives to maintain a relatively steady body temperature to operate optimally. Straying away from our setpoint temperature (approximately 98.6°F or 37°C) activates several feedback loops designed to increase or decrease our core body temperatures until we achieve the setpoint temperature again (we actually never truly achieve the setpoint temperature; our core temperature fluctuates around it). The effectiveness of the actions in these loops depends on the rate at which the tissues in our body store and transport heat. Therefore, to effectively replace a tissue or provide cells with an environment similar to their native tissue upon transplantation, tissue engineers must consider the heat transfer properties of the materials that they use. This is important in two ways: if an engineer is creating a tissue under culture conditions the materials in the scaffold must effectively allow the cells to receive the heat from the environment (incubator) and deliver any excess heat to the surrounding media. If the cell-seeded scaffold is being implanted, it must be able to effectively transfer excess heat away from the scaffold while maintaining a temperature needed for cell and tissue development.

There are three primary ways to transport heat: conduction, convection, and radiation. Heat transfer from conduction is the result of the collision of molecules. Higher energy molecules associated with a higher temperature collide with lower energy molecules associated with a lower temperature. In metallic materials, conduction also occurs through the transfer of free electrons. Convection is the transfer of heat through fluid flow. In convection, there is a transfer of energy between a surface and a fluid. Radiation is the transfer of heat without conduction or convection. The heat is transferred by electromagnetic waves between two surfaces.

Conduction can be described using Fourier's Law.

$$q_x = -Ak\frac{dT}{dx}$$

where q_x is the heat transfer rate in the x direction, A is the area normal to the direction of heat transfer, k is the thermal conductivity (which is unique to every material), and dT/dx is the change in temperature as a function of distance in the x direction. If we are measuring radial heat transfer through a tubular structure such as a blood vessel, the equation can be adapted to:

$$q_r = -Ak\frac{dT}{dr}$$

where q_r is the radial heat transfer rate and dT/dr is the change in temperature as a function of the distance radially.

Heat transfer as a result of convection can be found using the equation,

$$q = Ah\Delta T$$

where h is the heat transfer coefficient and ΔT is the temperature gradient. The heat transfer coefficient, h, depends on the geometry, nature of the fluid flow, and physical properties of the fluid. There are two types of convection: free convection and forced convection. In free convection (also called *natural convection*), the fluid is not flowing; it is next to a solid surface and there is heat circulation because of temperature differences throughout the fluid. In forced convection, a fluid is forced to flow past a solid surface because of an external force.

Heat transfer through radiation does not require a fluid. Energy is emitted from a solid; the heat transfer as a result of that radiation is given by,

$$q = A\sigma T^4$$

where, q is the emission rate of the radiating energy, A is the area that the energy is emitting from, σ is the Stefan-Boltzmann constant, and T is the absolute temperature.

PROBLEM 2.1

You are designing a material to be used as a regenerative covering for burn victims. Because temperature regulation is an important job for skin, the covering should have a similar thermal conductivity to skin. To measure the conductivity, you set up an experiment where one side of the material is 35°C and the other side is 20°C. The heat is flowing through that thickness of the material (2 mm) at a flux of 25 W/m². Assume that the properties of the material are constant throughout the volume, the heat is only flowing in the x direction and is moving at a steady state. Solve for the thermal conductivity.

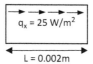

$q_x = 25$ W/m²

$L = 0.002$m

Remember:

$$q_x = -Ak\frac{dT}{dx}$$

We can rearrange it to:

$$k = -q_x \frac{1}{A}\frac{dx}{dT}$$

To simplify things, we can use the information in the problem. Because the flux is given in terms of area (m² in the denominator), we can say that $q_x(1/A)$ is 25 W/m². The term dx is just the change in length over which the heat transfer is occurring; so in our problem $dx = L$, 2 mm. The term dT is the measured change in temperature that occurs over dx; in our problem it is the difference between T_2 and T_1. Because the equation has a negative sign, we will make dT negative by taking the difference between T_1 and T_2. So then we can solve the following equation:

$$k = 25 \text{ W}/\text{m}^2 \frac{0.002 \text{ m}}{(35-20)^\circ\text{C}} = 3.33 \times 10^{-3} \text{ W}/\text{m}^2$$

2.3 MASS TRANSFER THROUGH DIFFUSION

Mass transfer is defined as the movement of a component from an area of high concentration to an area of lower concentration. Typically when we envision mass transfer in engineering, we think of the mixing of chemicals in a pipe or a vat, the blending of two powders in pharmaceuticals. In everyday life, examples include mixing sugar into our lemonade or stirring cream into our coffee. Mass transfer is also of great importance in the human body, and therefore, tissue engineering. Proteins, glucose, water, and ions are being moved into and out of the bloodstream to provide cells with the necessary nutrients to function optimally. Additionally carbon dioxide, ammonia, urea, and other wastes and metabolic by-products are moving into the bloodstream and out to be removed from the body by exhalation, urination, etc. So to sponsor cellular proliferation, cellular development, and tissue generation, scaffolding structures and their surrounding environments must facilitate tissue health by allowing for the efficient transport of nutrients and waste. The surrounding environment (media, blood, synovial fluid, interstitial liquid, etc.), material used in the scaffolds, and the structure of the scaffold must supply seeded cells with nutrients and aid in the removal of their waste in a way that is rapid and effective. Therefore, tissue engineers must take into consideration the abilities of nutrients and waste products to move throughout the volume by diffusion.

Diffusion occurs when a mixture of particles move within a solute from a place of higher concentration to a place of lower concentration. These particles can be solids, liquids, or gases. Diffusion can either be steady state or unsteady state. Steady-state diffusion takes place at a constant rate. The number of particles moving across the studied interface (the flux) is constant per unit time. So if you measure the change in concentration as you increase or decrease the distance from the interface (dc/dx), you obtain a constant, and if you measure a change in concentration as a function of a change in time (dc/dt), you get zero. In unsteady-state diffusion, the number of particles moving across the studied interface (the flux) is not constant per unit time; it changes with time. In this text, we will deal with steady-state diffusion.

The basic law governing the movement of particles is Fick's First Law. It can be written as

$$J_{A,x} = -D_{AB} \frac{dc_A}{dx}$$

where J_A is the molar flux in the x direction, D_{AB} is the diffusion coefficient of material A diffusing into material B, and dc_A/dx describes the change in the concentration of material A as you move in the x direction. According to this equation, we can adjust the rate that a species moves through our material by altering the concentration (c_A), altering the distance available to move through (x), or altering the diffusion constant (D_{AB}). We can control the diffusion coefficient by carefully selecting our scaffold material or the media surrounding the scaffold.

Therefore, the diffusion coefficient is extremely important for nutrient and waste diffusion, and therefore, the health of seeded cells. An increase in the diffusion coefficient means that the species can move through the material more quickly and a decrease in the diffusion coefficient means that the species moves through the material more slowly. Along with the chemistry of the material, the diffusion coefficient is affected by the pressure and temperature. The units for the diffusion coefficient are length^2/time. Diffusion coefficients for systems have been found experimentally or approximated mathematically.

Diffusion coefficients have been calculated for gases, liquids, and solids. It can be argued that because the majority of the weight in our tissues is because of water, we can estimate the diffusion coefficient of human tissues by using that of water (and the solute in question). Because we are trying to mimic the tissue environment in tissue engineering, we can use that same simplification. On the other hand, several researchers have calculated the diffusion coefficients of natural tissues and materials within an aqueous environment.

PROBLEM 2.2

Oxygen content is important for cell growth. Scaffolds must allow oxygen to reach the cells seeded inside. To test whether a scaffold is appropriate for use with cells, an experiment where the 2-mm thick scaffold is between two chambers is set up. The oxygen concentrations at each side of the scaffold are 0.25 kg/m³ and 2.1 kg/m³. Calculate the diffusion coefficient if the diffusion flux is 2.0×10^{-6} kg/m²-sec.

We can just plug the values into Fick's Law and solve for the coefficient.

$$J_{A,x} = -D_{AB} \frac{dc_A}{dx}$$

The flux, J, is 2.0×10^{-6} kg/m²-sec and dc_A/dx is the change in concentration, dc_A, (2.1–0.25 kg/m³) over the thickness of the scaffold, dx, (2 mm or 0.002 m).

$$2 \times 10^{-6} \frac{\text{kg}}{\text{m}^2 \text{sec}} = -D_{AB} \frac{\left(0.25 \frac{\text{kg}}{\text{m}^3} - 2.1 \frac{\text{kg}}{\text{m}^3} \right)}{0.002 \, \text{m}}$$

$$2.16 \times 10^9 \frac{\text{m}^2}{\text{sec}} = D_{AB}$$

It can be argued that the solute molecules are actually moving within the solvent (typically water) that has been absorbed by the scaffold. Therefore, the chemistry of the material, specifically the hydrophobicity or hydrophilicity, can affect the diffusion coefficient by affecting the amount of liquid that penetrates the matrix. If the scaffold material is more hydrophilic, it can absorb more water and make the transport of solutes easier in an aqueous environment. If it is more hydrophobic, less water penetrates the matrix, making the transport of solutes more difficult. The material can also affect the diffusion coefficient based on the solute. The charge-charge interactions between the matrix and the solute, for example, could drastically affect the diffusion coefficient.

The porosity of the matrix also has an effect on the diffusion coefficient. This is related to the previous simplification about transport mainly taking place in the water absorbed by the matrix. If this is the case, then water will flow more freely in pores than inside of the matrix material. So the porosity of a matrix presents a unique issue because molecular transport occurs in the solute inside of the pores but is hindered by the matrix material along the pore wall. So increased pore diameter will positively affect the diffusion coefficient, whereas a decreased diameter will negatively affect it. This process is called *hindered diffusion* and can be accounted for using the following equation:

$$D_{Ae} = D_{AB}^{\circ} F_1(\varphi) F_2(\varphi)$$

D_{AB}° is the molecular diffusion coefficient of A (solute) in B (solvent) at infinite dilution. $F_1(\varphi)$ is a correctional factor based on the relationship between the pore diameter and the solute molecular diameter. It is found using the following equation:

$$F_1(\varphi) = \frac{\pi \left(d_{pore} - d_s \right)^2}{\pi d_{pore}^2} = \frac{\text{solute flux area}}{\text{total flux area}} = (1-\varphi)^2$$

In this equation, φ is found using the equation,

$$\varphi = \frac{\text{solute molecular diameter, } d_s}{\text{pore diameter, } d_{pore}}$$

and $F_2(\varphi)$ is the hydrodynamic hindrance factor; it is based on the hindrance of solute Brownian motion within the pores. There are several different ways to calculate the hindrance factor based on pore shapes, particle drag, and particle size. The most commonly used equation is the Renkin equation. This equation assumes the presence of cylindrical pores.

$$F_2(\varphi) = (1-\varphi)^2 \left(1 - 2.104\varphi + 2.09\varphi^3 - 0.95\varphi^5 \right)$$

When the pore diameter is much larger than the solute diameter, the equation simplifies to:

$$F_2(\varphi) = \left(1 - 2.104\varphi + 2.09\varphi^3 - 0.95\varphi^5 \right)$$

Each of these factors, $F_1(\varphi)$ and $F_2(\varphi)$, range from 0 to 1 and serve to reduce the diffusion coefficient, D_{AB}°, acknowledging that the presence of the matrix inhibits movement of the solute through the solvent.

PROBLEM 2.3
You are building a scaffold for tissue engineering and are deciding on the appropriate pore size. The technique that you are currently using creates an average pore size of 250 nm. There is another technique that would create pore sizes of 500 nm, but it is much more expensive. To see if it is worth increasing the pore size, you decide to calculate the difference in the diffusion coefficient of oxygen in the scaffold and media with both types of pores. If the diffusion coefficient with the 500 nm pores is at least 20% larger than the coefficient for the 250 nm pores for both gases, you will use the larger pores. Based on your calculations should you use the scaffold with the larger pores?

The diameter for oxygen is 3.0 Å (Modern Physics, D. Freude). The diffusion coefficient for oxygen is 3.24×10^{-5} cm²/s.[3]

To solve this problem we do not need to solve for the actual diffusion constant, D_{AB}, we just need to find if the ratio of D_{AB} to D_{AB}° shows an increase of at least 20%. Because we have the pore sizes and molecular diameters, we can solve for φ, plug it into the equations for F_1 and F_2 and then see the relationship between D_{AB} and D_{AB}°.

For the 250 nm pores:

$$\varphi = \frac{3 \text{ Angstroms}}{250 \text{ nm}} = \frac{3 \times 10^{-10}}{25 \times 10^{-10}} = 0.12$$

Now plug this into the equations for F_1 and F_2.

$$F_1(\varphi) = (1-\varphi)^2 = (1-0.12)^2 = 0.774$$

Because 25 is not a lot larger than 3 we will use the first equation for F_2.

$$F_2(\varphi) = (1-0.12)^2 (1-2.104(0.12)+2.09(0.12)^3 -0.95(0.12)^5)$$

$$F_2(\varphi) = 0.774(0.748+0.004-2.4 \times 10^{-5}) = 0.582$$

Now plug these values into the equation for hindered diffusion through the 250-nm scaffold.

$$D_{Ae} = 3.2 \times 10^{-5} \frac{\text{cm}^2}{\text{sec}} (0.774)(0.582) = 1.44 \times 10^{-5} \frac{\text{cm}^2}{\text{sec}}$$

or

$$D_{Ae} = D_{AB}^{\circ}(0.774)(0.582) = 0.45 \, D_{AB}^{\circ}$$

Now we repeat these calculations for 500 nm

$$\varphi = \frac{3 \text{ Angstroms}}{500 \text{ nm}} = \frac{3 \times 10^{-10}}{50 \times 10^{-10}} = 0.06$$

Now plug this into the equations for F_1 and F_2.

$$F_1(\varphi) = (1-\varphi)^2 = (1-0.06)^2 = 0.884$$

Because 50 is not a lot larger than 3 we will use the first equation for F_2.

$$F_2(\varphi) = (1-0.06)^2 (1-2.104(0.06)+2.09(0.06)^3 -0.95(0.06)^5)$$

$$F_2(\varphi) = 0.884(0.873+4.5 \times 10^{-4} -7.4 \times 10^{-7}) = 0.772$$

Now plug these values into the equation for hindered diffusion through the 500-nm pore scaffold.

$$D_{Ae} = 3.2 \times 10^{-5} \frac{cm^2}{sec} (0.884)(0.772) = 2.18 \times 10^{-5} \frac{cm^2}{sec}$$

or

$$D_{Ae} = D_{AB}^{\circ} (0.884)(0.772) = 0.68 D_{AB}^{\circ}$$

The difference between $0.45\ D_{AB}$ and $0.68\ D_{AB}$ is 0.23, greater than 20% so you should use the scaffold with the 500-nm pores.

2.4 IMPORTANCE TO TISSUE ENGINEERING

Although in many calculations we make the assumption that the temperature of the human body is steady at 37°C, in actuality its temperature fluctuates throughout the day. Fluctuations may be caused by external temperature, sickness, or exercise. Therefore, the tissues in the body must have heat transfer coefficients that allow the body to efficiently generate and give off heat to warm up or lose heat at the correct rate to cool down. If the heat transfer coefficients of these tissues and fluids allow them to hold on to heat for too long or remove heat too quickly, cell and tissue death are real possibilities. If we are designing tissue replacements for implantation, the materials that we use should have similar heat transfer coefficients to the tissues that they are replacing. Otherwise this may cause that part of the body to retain too much heat or hold on to too much heat, potentially causing cell and tissue damage.

Similar to heat transfer, diffusion is an extremely important concept in tissue engineering. The diffusion of ions, nutrients, and waste products is extremely important for cellular health and eventual tissue regeneration. Oxygen and carbon dioxide must move freely through the scaffold to reach cells implanted in the cells. Nutrients from the surrounding media must be able to reach all cells seeded throughout the scaffold thickness. For the cells to receive nutrients and for the waste to move far from the cells, the diffusion coefficients of these molecules with the material in the scaffold must be sufficiently large. If the diffusion coefficients are too small, the cells in the center of the scaffold may be starved and die. This creates a "hollowing out" of the scaffold, sometimes referred to as a *necrotic core*. The scaffold develops tissue along the surface, but further in (where the nutrients can't reach the cells by diffusion), there is no tissue growth because of cell death.

Another area where diffusion coefficients are of huge consequence in tissue engineering is the use of growth factors and other biomolecules to enhance tissue growth and development within a scaffold. A commonly used way to introduce growth factors to cells is to elute them from implanted scaffolds. The scaffolds may be soaked in a growth factor solution prior to implantation or the scaffold could be formed with the growth factor inside of the polymer solution before the scaffold is made. In either case the diffusivity coefficient of the material, scaffold porosity, and growth factor are important for obtaining a release rate for the growth factor that best aids cell and tissue growth and development. Typically, researchers want to avoid the quick release of all of the growth factor and prefer a slow, sustained release.

QUESTIONS

1. The inner and outer temperature of a polymeric membrane with a thermal conductivity of 0.7 W/mK are 37.5°C and 35°C, respectively. The sample has a height, width, and thickness of 20, 10, and 1.5 mm, respectively. Assuming that heat is only traveling through the material perpendicular to the thickness, how much heat is being lost?

2. The inner and outer temperatures of a 5-mm thick cardiac muscle graft in a special twin bath culture system are 37°C and 27°C, respectively. What is the heat loss from a section that is 2 mm in width and 3 mm in length if the thermal conductivity of the graft is 0.25 W/mK? Assume that the properties of the material are constant throughout the volume, the heat is only flowing in the x direction, and is moving at a steady state.

3. You are developing an artificial skin graft that has a heat insulating covering to allow the patient to leave the hospital after implantation without suffering from debilitating heat loss or overheating. You set up a test where the covering and underlying graft are at 35°C and the air surrounding them is room temperature, 20°C. If your heat transfer coefficient under these circumstances is 7.5 W/m²K, how much heat is leaving the surface through convection?

4. You make some changes to the skin substitute do that the thermal conductivity of the material is 1.8 W/mK, and now you would like to find the rate of heat lost through it. You set it up so that the inner side is at 20°C and the outer side is at 37°C. The material is 2-mm thick with a width of 1 cm and length of 3 cm. Assume one-dimensional conduction in the x direction, steady-state conditions, and uniform properties throughout the material.

5. You have developed a device to add additional oxygen to your media (solution that you add to nourish the cells in cell culture). You essentially blow oxygen rich air over the media and then collect it. Unfortunately, you cannot warm the air before you introduce it to the media, so it is introduced at 20°C and the media is 37°C. How much heat is lost by convection of the heat transfer coefficient between the media surface and the air is 30 W/m²K?

6. You formed a company based on the technology from the previous question and now mass produce the engineered tissues. You now have a system that simultaneously oxygenates the cell media and maintains its temperature at 37°C by blowing warm heavily oxygenated air over it. Unfortunately, today the system has broken and is blowing the air at room temperature, 20°C. How much heat is leaving the liquid surface (heat flux) if the heat transfer coefficient under these conditions is 35 W/m² K? If the unit were to stop blowing the room temperature air, how much heat would leave the media if the media has a thermal conductivity of 0.610 W/m K?

7. Cells have been seeded inside of a hydrogel submerged in media. Above the hydrogel, the well is filled with media (dimensions of 1 cm × 1 cm × 0.5 cm). The cells are

producing CO_2 creating a concentration in the hydrogel of 35 mg/m^3. When added to the hydrogel, the media had a CO_2 concentration of 5 mg/m^3. If the diffusion coefficient is 0.25 m^2/min, what is the CO_2 flux from the hydrogel to the media?

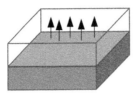

8. A thin polymeric scaffold is placed on top of a hydrogel and submitted into media. The hydrogel is initially oxygen poor, whereas the media is oxygen rich. If a steady state of oxygen diffusion is achieved, calculate the diffusion flux of oxygen through the polymeric scaffold if the diffusion coefficient is 5×10^{-10} m^2/s concentrations of oxygen at 2.5 and 5 mm beneath the polymeric scaffold are 2.0 and 2.4 kg/m^3, respectively?

9. The same setup is used again. The thin polymeric scaffold has a thickness of 1 mm. When steady state is reached, the oxygen concentrations are measured at 0.02 and 0.055 wt%. What is the diffusion coefficient if the flux is 3.4×10^{-8} kg/m^3?

10. You are building a scaffold for a cell type that extremely active. Because of their level of activity, they must receive enough oxygen but also be able to clear carbon dioxide in an efficient manner. To ensure the survival of the cells, you must design a scaffold with pore sizes that are large enough to cause the hindered diffusion coefficients of oxygen and carbon dioxide to be no less than 70% of the normal coefficients. What is the minimal pore size that accomplishes this for both gases? The diameters for oxygen and carbon dioxide are 3.0 and 3.4 Å, respectively (Modern Physics, D. Freude). The diffusion coefficients for oxygen and carbon dioxide in the normal are 3.24 and 2.41 cm^2/s, respectively.[3]

REFERENCES

1. Deen WM. *Analysis of Transport Phenomena*. 2nd ed. New York: Oxford University Press; 2012.
2. Welty JR, Wicks CE et al. *Fundamentals of Momentum, Heat, and Mass Transfer*. 5th ed. Hoboken, NJ: John Wiley & Sons; 2008.
3. Richard T. Calculating the oxygen diffusion coefficient in water. http://compost.css.cornell.edu/oxygen/oxygen.diff.water.html.

CHAPTER 3

Biomolecules and Tissue Properties

3.1 INTRODUCTION

The behavior and function of a tissue is dictated by its composition and its architecture. The molecules present in the tissue combined with their arrangement in the tissue give it specific properties (mechanical, electrical, etc.). In this chapter, we will review some biomacromolecules that are present in a wide range of tissues and then discuss how they contribute to the function of several types of tissues. We will focus on two types of organic molecules (proteins and proteoglycans) and one type of inorganic molecule biological mineral (calcium phosphate). In each section, we will discuss basic characteristics and then give examples that are important to tissue function and structure.

3.2 PROTEINS

Proteins are long polymer chains made of smaller repeating molecules (monomers) called *amino acids* (Figures 3.1 and 3.2). Small numbers of amino acids combine to form polypeptides (Figure 3.1), which then combine to form proteins. All amino acids have the same basic structure; the differences between them lie in their side groups (R groups). There are 20 different R groups, 18 are side chains, 1 is a hydrogen atom, and 1 is a proline ring (Figure 3.2). The R groups determine the shape, properties, and function of proteins based on their size and chemistry. Each protein has an N terminal end (the part of the protein that terminates with a NH_2, also called *amino group*) and a C terminal end (the part of the protein that terminates with the COOH, also called *carboxyl group*).

Proteins have multiple layers of structure; they are primary, secondary, tertiary, and quaternary structures. The primary structure is the amino acid sequence of the polypeptide. It is the list of amino acids in the protein in order. The secondary structure is the

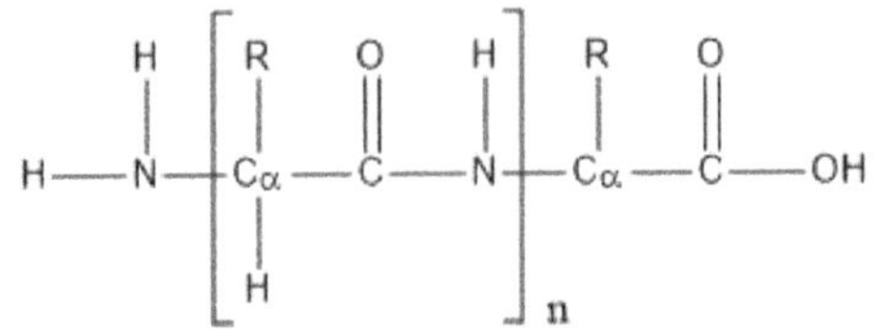

FIGURE 3.1 Polypeptide chemical formula.

three-dimensional shape that results after the folding of a chain or part of a chain. It is regular, repeated patterns of folding of the protein backbone. The folding is the result of the interactions between the amino acids in the primary structure. The forces that drive protein folding are hydrophobicity and hydrophilicity. To hide hydrophobic side chains, molecules fold in different ways creating commonly used motifs (the two most common folding patterns are the alpha helix and the beta sheet). Proteins fold in a way that packs hydrophobic side chains into the interior of the molecule. This makes a hydrophilic shell and hydrophobic core (Figures 3.3 and 3.4).

The tertiary structure is formed by packing the motifs from the secondary structure into one or several domains. So the tertiary structure is the result of multiple motifs in one amino acid chain interacting with each other. The tertiary structure is held together by disulfide bonds, ionic bonds, hydrogen bonds, hydrophobic interactions, and hydrophilic interactions.

The quaternary structure is the organization that results from interactions between different chains. In the final protein, several polypeptide chains (tertiary structures) are arranged into a quaternary structure. Important quaternary structures include collagen, hemoglobin, and laminin.

3.2.1 Collagen

Collagen is a major structural protein in vertebrates. It is the basic structural element in hard and soft tissues and is a major component of extracellular matrices (ECMs). Collagen forms the essential mechanical building blocks in the musculoskeletal system. It is present in most of the connective and supportive tissues in vertebrates and makes up almost 30% of all protein in the human body. Presently at least 26 types of collagen have been identified, and additional collagens have been found in invertebrates (Figure 3.5).

Collagen has great tensile strength, acting as the main component of cartilage, ligaments, tendons, bone, and teeth. Along with keratin, it is responsible for skin strength and elasticity. Its degradation leads to wrinkles that accompany aging. Collagen also strengthens blood vessels and is present in the cornea and lens of the eye. Collagen is the main load-bearing element in blood vessels, skin, tendons, bone, ligament, cornea, fascia, dura matter, etc.

The basic structure of collagen is a triple helix that consists of three left-handed helices that are wound into a right handed triple helix (Figure 3.5). It looks like a coiled-coil.

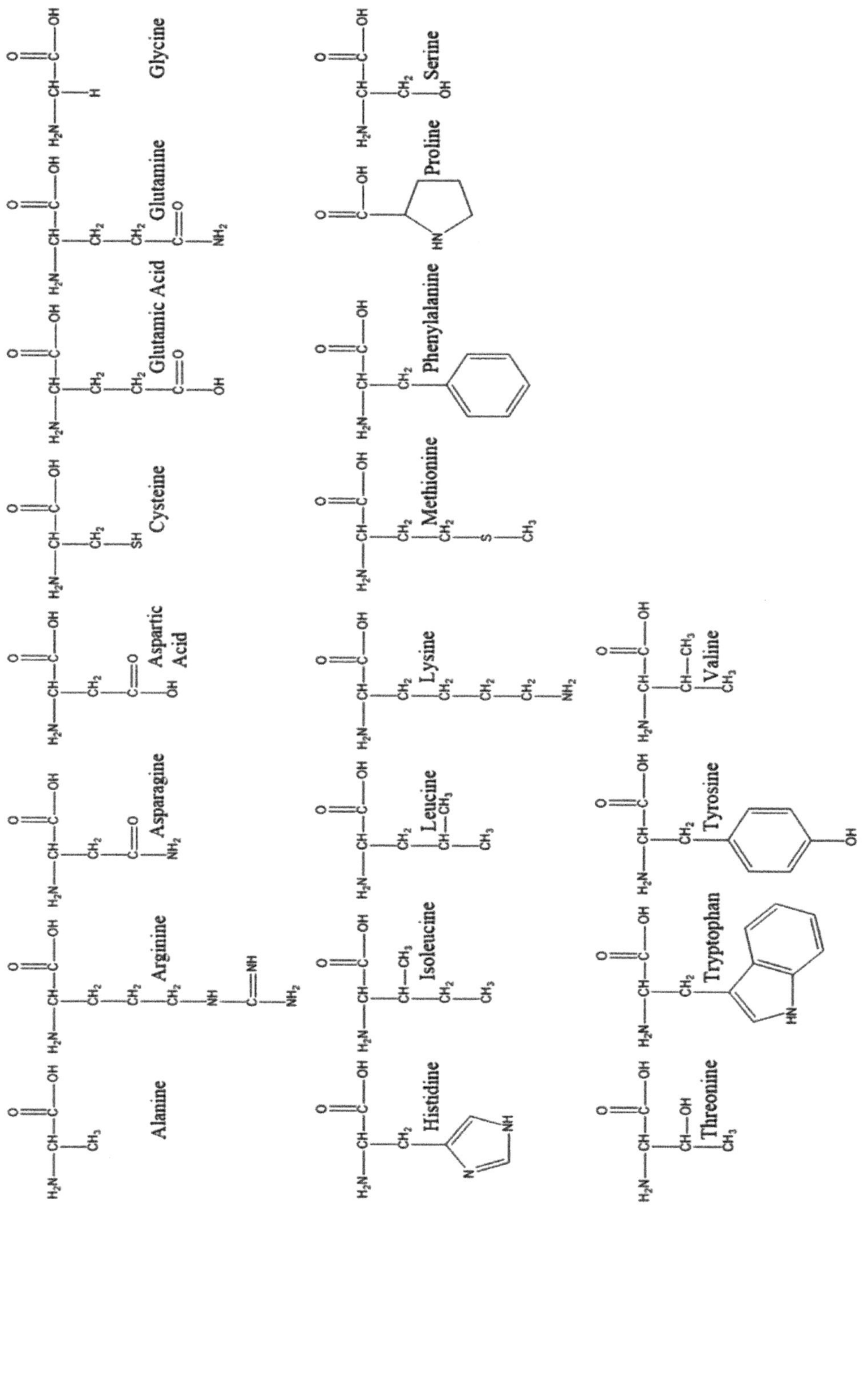

FIGURE 3.2   Chemical formulas of amino acids with different R groups.

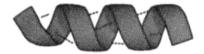

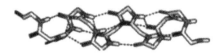

FIGURE 3.3   Alpha helix from Wikipedia and the Protein Data Bank.

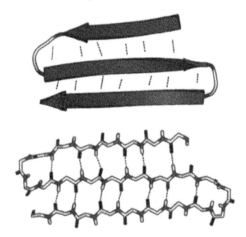

FIGURE 3.4   Beta sheet from Wikipedia and the Protein Data Bank.

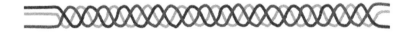

FIGURE 3.5   Illustration of the collagen triple helix.

The side chains point away from the triple helix and can contact neighboring molecules for better packing. The basic unit of collagen is the alpha-chain (α-chain). Collagen is a rod-like molecule, approximately 300 nm long and 1.5 nm in diameter. Individual chains are also referred to as *polyproline II helices*.

The triple helix is a right-handed coiled coil and a cooperative quaternary structure stabilized by numerous hydrogen bonds. These chains contain multiple repeats of the amino acid sequence Gly-X-Y, where X and Y are usually proline or hydroxyproline. Of all of the amino acids in the molecule, 33% of them are glycine, and 25% are proline and hydroxyproline. Type I collagen contains 2 αI chains and 1 αII chain. Collagens can be split into two major groups: fiber forming and non-fiber forming. Type I collagen is the most abundant, found in skin, bones, tendons, and ligaments. Type II collagen is the major cartilage collagen, found in cartilage, nucleus pulposus (spine), and vitreous humor (eye). Type III collagen is located in granulation tissue in pliable tissues such as blood vessels, skin (in reticular fiber), uterus, and intestines. Type IV collagen is found in all basement membranes, eye lens, and the kidney. Type V collagen is a minor component in most interstitial tissues and placenta. Type IX collagen is a minor component in hyaline cartilage. Type X collagen is located in mineralizing cartilage, acting as a minor component in hyaline cartilage and ligament. Type XI collagen is found in cartilage, and Type XII collagen is found on the surface of collagen fibrils and may connect fibrillar collagens to other components of the ECM. Collagen I, II, and III are the major types of collagen (responsible for prevention of failure because of tensile and shear forces). Others collagen types are found in small amounts.

3.2.1.1 Collagen: Structure

The types I, II, and III collagen molecules are triple helices composed of three left-handed polyproline II helices intertwined in a right-handed manner. The triple helix is approximately 300 nm long and 1.5 nm wide with about 1000 amino acids per chain. The triple helix has a rise per residue of 2.9 angstroms, with 3.3 residues per turn and a rise per turn of 9.6 angstroms. In the triple helix, the three chains are held together by direct hydrogen bonding between proline C=O groups on one chain and glycine NH groups on another, as well as water-mediated bonds where the triple helix is disrupted, and water infiltrates the structure. The three chains are also held together by direct and water-mediated hydrogen bonding in collagen (Figure 3.6).

Studies involving molecular modeling and the production of triple helical polypeptides have shown that changes in the glycine–proline–hydroxyproline repeat alter the appearance and stability of the triple helix. The triple helix requires glycine to be present every third amino acid because it is the only amino acid small enough to be in the center of the super helix. Proline and hydroxyproline play important roles in the stability of the collagen triple helix, stabilizing structurally and thermally. The absence of these amino acids has been shown to cause a disruption in the collagen triple helix.

The ring in the backbone forces the polypeptide to turn and limits mobility. Ringed amino acids have limited degrees of freedom. Their removal causes conformational changes that create a local untwisting of the triple helix, giving the area more conformational freedom. Conformational plots have shown that repeats without PRO and HYP have

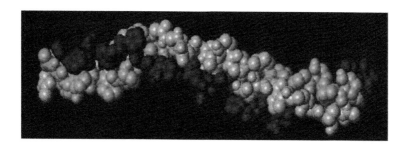

FIGURE 3.6 Molecular model of a section of the collagen type I triple helix that lacks the GLY-PRO-HYP repeat.

greater conformational freedom. Molecular modeling experiments have shown that these areas may be more flexible than GLY-PRO-HYP repeat.

There may be flexible and rigid regions in the collagen molecule and microfibril. These regions contribute to the mechanical behavior of collagenous tissues. Collagen fibrils also contain 12 bands that appear after positive staining with solutions of heavy metal ions. The bands are labeled a1, a2, a3, a4, b1, b2, c1, c2, c3, d, e1, and e2).

3.2.1.2 Collagen: Synthesis

Collagens are synthesized within cells in a precursor form termed *procollagen*. This has amino (N) and carboxyl (C) terminal non-helical ends that are about 15.0 and 10.0 nm long, respectively. Figure 3.7 is a diagram of procollagen type I molecule with amino pro-peptides (left-hand portion of molecule), an amino non-helical end (straight portion), a triple helical region, a carboxylic non-helical end, and a carboxylic propeptide (right-hand end of molecule). The amino (N-) and carboxylic (C-) propeptides are cleaved by specific proteases during collagen self-assembly.

The presence of amino (N) and carboxylic terminal (C) extensions on the collagen molecule have been shown to limit self-assembly of procollagen to about five molecules. Removal of the N- and C-propeptides by specific proteinases occurs prior to final fibril assembly. The C-propeptides are essential for both the initiation of procollagen molecular assembly from the constituent chains and lateral assembly of procollagen molecules. Results of studies on embryonic skin suggest that the N-propeptides remain attached to fibrils 20–30 nm in diameter after collagen is assembled. The N-propeptide is removed before further lateral fibril growth occurs. After the C-propeptide is cleaved, fibril diameters appear to increase, suggesting that the C-propeptide is associated with initiation of fibrillogenesis.

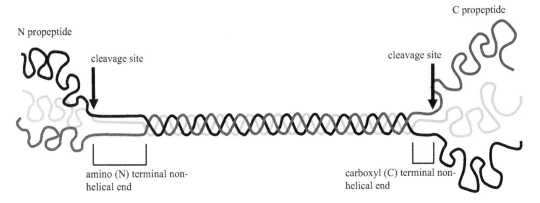

FIGURE 3.7   Drawing of tropocollagen including cleavage sites, N- and C-propeptides, and N- and C-nonhelical ends.

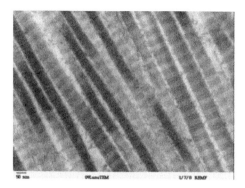

FIGURE 3.8   Transmission electron microscope (TEM) image of collagen fibers from lung tissue by Louisa Howard from http://remf.dartmouth.edu/imagesindex.html and https://commons.wikimedia.org/wiki/File:Fibers_of_Collagen_Type_I_-_TEM.jpg.

3.2.1.3 Collagen: Fibril Assembly

There are several fibril-forming collagens (most prominent I, II, and III). All of the fibril-forming collagens self-assemble into cross-striated fibrils with a characteristic 67 nm repeat; they all share a triple helical region that is roughly 1000 amino acid residues long with a length of about 300 nm. This is called a "quarter-staggered" packing pattern. Fiber-forming collagens self-assemble to form microfibrils, fibrils, and fibers. Other organizational units vary from tissue to tissue. Type I collagen self-assembles *in vivo* to form a quarter-staggered array of molecules that are staggered by about 22% of their length with respect to their nearest neighbor. This appears as a striation pattern in electron micrographs (seen in tendon and skin; Figure 3.8).

Collagen molecules self-assemble by a combination of linear and lateral aggregation. Initial linear and lateral aggregation are promoted by the presence of both the N- and C-propeptides. When both propeptides are intact, lateral assembly is limited and the fibrils are narrow (Figure 3.9). Removal of the N-propeptides results in lateral assembly of narrow fibrils. The subsequent removal of the C-propeptides results in additional lateral growth of fibrils.[1]

When type I collagen molecules are self-assembled into a quarter-staggered array, two distinct regions, the overlap and gap (also called *hole*), can be identified in negatively stained collagenous tissues in the electron microscope (overlap region and gap region; Figure 3.10).

The overlap region is 20 nm in length and the gap region is 47 nm long; all of these regions are repeated throughout the tissue. The periodic length of the striation is termed "D." This length is the staggered distance; it varies from tissue to tissue depending on the molecular tilt angle. The distance D is 65 nm in skin, 67 nm in tendon, 64 nm in native fibrils, and 68 nm in moistened fibrils. The length of each molecule is 4.4 times that of the period of striation "D," so each molecule is 4.4 D long with a 0.6 D gap between molecule ends. If you're doing the math in your head … 67 nm × 4.4 = 268 nm which is approximately 300 nm, the length of a collagen molecule.

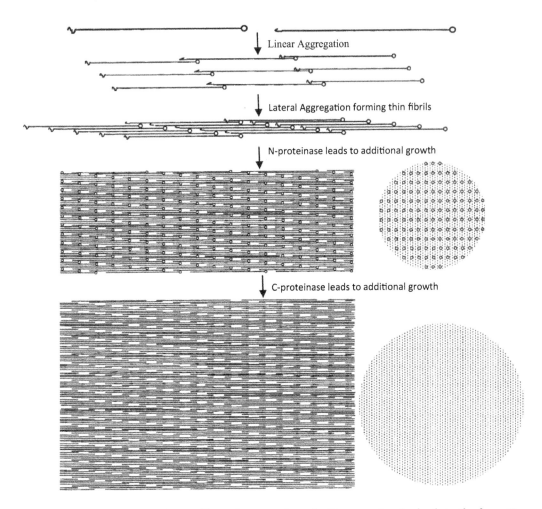

FIGURE 3.9 Linear aggregation and lateral aggregation of collagen molecules leads to the formation of fibril sheets. The procollagen molecule is represented by a straight line with bent (N-propeptide) and circular (C-propeptide) regions. Their arrangement leads to overlap and gap regions that create a striated appearance in the fibers and tissues. (From Silver, F.H. et al., *J. Biomech.*, 36, 1529–1553, 2003.)

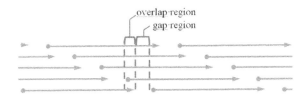

FIGURE 3.10 Overlap and gap regions for collage self-assembly.

Collagen self-assembles through direct hydrogen bonds and water-mediated hydrogen bonds. The amino acid side chains and glycine C=O groups come into contact with neighboring NH groups and water molecules outside of the triple helix. As stated, these water molecules contact the hydroxyl groups of HYP and C=O and NH groups of amino acids in neighboring molecules. This occurs inside of the molecule as well.

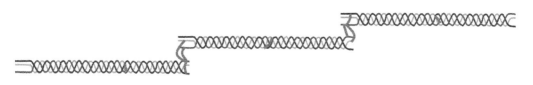

FIGURE 3.11 Schematic of intramolecular crosslinks (within the same collagen molecule) and intermolecular crosslinks (between neighboring collagen molecules). (Based off of a figure from Medscape.com.)

3.2.1.4 Collagen: Properties

Type I collagen fibers have an elastic modulus of 5–900 MPa and a ultimate tensile strength (UTS) of 2–92 MPa.[2,3] Collagenous tissues increase in strength with the development of crosslinks, which stabilize collagen fibers. The formation of these crosslinks involves histidine, lysine, and hydroxylysine residues (Figure 3.11).

3.2.1.5 Collagen: Crosslinks

Along with hydrogen bonding, the strength of the collagen fibers depends on the formation of covalent crosslinks. Crosslinks occur between the telopeptide and adjacent helical domains of collagen molecules. Type I collagen has four cross-linking sites: one in each telopeptide and two others at the sites in the triple-helical domain at residues 87 and 930. Note that the position of intra- and intermolecular crosslinks causes increases in cross-linking change and collagenous tissue mechanical properties. Namely, it increases elastic modulus, increases UTS, and decreases strain to failure.

Defects in collagen cross-linking lead to severe diseases, including Ehlers-Danlos syndrome, Marfan syndrome, Menke's disease, and Cutis laxa (or you could say that severe diseases lead to cross-linking problems.) *In vivo* crosslinks are formed by the enzyme lysyl oxidase. The cross-linking is based on aldehyde formation from the single telopeptide lysine or hydroxylysine residues. Lysyl oxidase deaminates them, binding to the sequence (HylGly-His-Arg) opposite the N- and C-terminals of an adjacent quarter-staggered molecule. This reaction places stable crosslinks within (intramolecular crosslinks) and between the molecules (intermolecular crosslinks; Figure 3.12.

There are two types of crosslinks: allysine, the lysine derived aldehyde seen mainly in skin, cornea, and sclera, and hydroxyallysine, the hydroxylysine-derived aldehyde seen mainly in bone, cartilage, ligaments, and tendons. These crosslinks change over time, going from immature divalent crosslinks to mature trivalent crosslinks (Figure 3.13).

In addition to cross-linking by lysyl oxidase, collagens are also susceptible over time to further cross-linking through other reactions, namely with reducing sugars, usually glucose, and lipid oxidation products. *In vitro* crosslinks can also form in air through dehydration, dehydrothermal (DHT) crosslinking. DHT involves the removal of residual water and formation of synthetic peptide bonds. This is usually done in a vacuum oven above 90°C. DHT forms intermolecular crosslinks through condensation reactions either by esterification of carbonyl groups or amide formation (acetylation of amine groups). DHT enhances thermal stability and prevents denaturing at lower temperatures by decreasing the number of readily available positively and negatively charged amino acids.

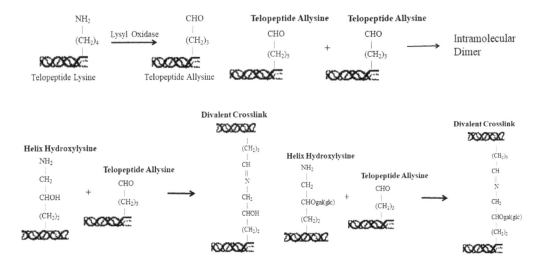

FIGURE 3.12   Schematic of immature crosslink formation.

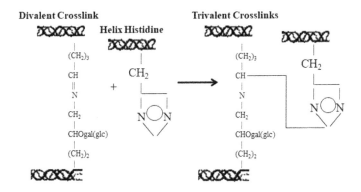

FIGURE 3.13   Schematic of mature crosslink formation.

3.2.1.6 Collagen: Mineralization

Calcium phosphate makes up a majority of the mineral present in bone and other hard tissues. (Hydroxyapatite, $Ca_{10}(PO_4)_6(OH)_2$). Crystal nucleation occurs first in the gap region (specifically in the e band), and then spreads onto overlap region of type I collagen. Gaps are three dimensional. Crystal nucleation in a collagenous matrix involves mineralization of a collagenous tissue, which causes increased UTS, increased elastic modulus, and decreased strain to failure.[4,5]

3.2.1.7 Collagen: Diseased States

Collagen diseases arise from genetic defects that affect the biosynthesis, assembly, posttranslational modification, secretion, or other processes in the normal production of collagen. Osteogenesis imperfecta (OI) is a brittle bone disease. This results from decreased quantity or quality of collagen I in the bone. Osteogenesis imperfect occurs when changes in certain amino acids in the triple helix affect collagen structure and assembly. This effects the nucleation and laying down of hydroxyapatite. In general, type I is the mildest form of this disease, whereas types IV, III, and II indicate increasing severities of disease. Aside from Type I, the life expectancy of patients with all other forms of OI is often assumed to be shortened. However, life expectancy of patients with OI type IA is the same as that of the general population. In type IB, mortality is modestly increased compared with that of the general population. Type II OI is fatal in the perinatal period, shortly before and after birth. Type III affects life expectancy; however, patients with type III OI surviving beyond the age of 10 years have a better outlook than other patients with OI. For Type IV, mortality is modestly increased compared with that of the general population.[6,7]

Another disease, Ehlers-Danlos syndrome (EDS), is a group of rare genetic disorders caused by a defect in collagen synthesis, varying from mild to life-threatening. EDS is caused by the partial cleavage of the N-propeptide. This allows the N-propeptide to become incorporated within the body of the fibrils. N-propeptides are in a bent-back conformation that is within the overlap region. There can be intact N-propeptides on fibril surfaces in type VII EDS, which alters fibrilogenesis and fiber packing. Common symptoms of EDS include unstable, flexible joints with a tendency to dislocate, ligaments which are overly stretchable, and elastic, fragile, soft skin that easily forms welts and scars. EDS can also affect bones and cause fragile blood vessels and organs.

Dermatosparaxis is a form of EDS that causes fragile skin. Fibrillogenesis of type I collagen is specifically impaired in the skin. In this disease, the N-propeptide of a chain is not cleaved. In some studies, 57% of the collagen molecules have intact N-propeptides, whose presence alters fibrilogenesis and fibril packing (prevents tight packing), resulting in skin that is easily torn.

3.2.1.8 Collagen: Types

There are at least 26 different types of collagen, which can be split in a number of different ways. Sorting by classes yields three groups: class 1, with a 300-nm triple helix; class 2, found in basement membranes; and class 3, which consists of short-chained molecules. Another method of classifying collagens is through types. Types I, II, and III are the major fibrillar collagens, whereas Types V, VI, IX, X, and XI, for instance, are other fibrillar collagens that are not found in as great a quantity as types I, II, and III. Fibril-associated collagens include VII, XII, XV, XVI, XIX, and XXI. Basement membrane collagens include IV and VIII.

Types I, II, and III are examples of collagens that form fibers. These molecules comprise microfibrils, which make up fibrils, which make up fibers, which form tissues. These are large load-bearing fibrillar collagens. That does not mean that these molecules don't associate; they also form various structures *in vivo*.

Nonfibrillar collagens do not form fibers. Nonfibrillar collagens can associate with fibrillar collagens. They may also associate with each other to form microfibrillar networks. These collagens have triple helical segments separated by larger noncollagenous sections. Triple helical segments vary in length. These collagens serve a variety of functions in different tissues or organs.

Type IV collagen is found in all tissue basement membranes, eye lens, and the kidney. Type IV forms networks by dimerization of the C-globular ends, formation of tetramers through parallel and anti-parallel alignment at the N-terminal triple helical segments, as well as forming sheetlike structures.

Type V collagen is a minor component in most interstitial tissues, placenta, tendon, skin, and cardiovascular tissue. It forms a matrix around cells. Type V forms associations with type I and type III collagen. Type V is in the core, type III forms the outer layer, and type I associates with the outer layer.

Type VI collagen is found in the ECMs of cardiovascular tissue, placenta, ligaments, tendons, uterus, skin, and cornea. It forms microfibrillar meshes composed of microfibrils that assemble end to end. Microfibrils have a 100-nm periodicity and are composed of alternating globular and filamentous portions.

Type VII collagen is present in skin. Its molecules assemble into short filaments, which anchor the basement membrane to the dermal layer in skin.

Type VIII collagen is present in cardiovascular tissue and is found in sheetlike structures around endothelial cells.

Type IX collagen is a minor component in hyaline cartilage.

Type X collagen is in mineralizing cartilage, acting as a minor component in hyaline cartilage and ligament. Type X forms in sheetlike structures.

Type XI collagen is found in cartilage. This collagen is associated with striated type II fibrils in cartilage.

Type XII collagen is found on the surface of collagen fibrils and may connect fibrillar collagens to other components of the ECM. Their structure and resulting associations and structures allow the smaller fibrillar and nonfibrillar collagens to have different functions in different tissues. They form bonds between ECM components and add to the mechanical properties of the ECM.

These "minor" collagens can associate with other macromolecules in the ECM. They specifically can attach to other macromolecules that are important for tissue function (proteoglycans) and keep these macromolecules in the matrix. As a result, "minor" collagens maintain tissue structure. These collagens have bonding sites for cells. Some of the noncollagenous sequences include sections with amino acid sequences for fibronectin, a cell-adhesive glycoprotein that keeps cells attached to ECM, possibly transferring load to cell membrane through stretching.

Minor collagens form structural links, like glue between major structural molecules. They connect different parts of tissues, from the basement membrane to upper layers. These collagens also add to tissue elasticity and are found in flexible, soft tissues. These tissues undergo a great deal of repeated tensile stress. One type, uniaxial stress occurs in tendons and ligaments. Multiaxial stress occurs in the placenta, uterus, and skin.

Molecule to molecule and molecules to cell connections must be flexible. They prevent tissue and cell damage and transfer stress to cell membranes to alter cell behavior. These collagens form networks that are flexible or isotropic. In type VI, microfibrils link rods with globular sections and have flexibility in the globular sections.

Microfibrillar networks can transfer load in many different directions. In Type IV, networks are formed without a primary axis of orientation, so links between macromolecules are maintained under a variety of stress conditions. These collagens are found in tissues that experience frequent tensile stresses. Notable tissues include the kidney, eye lens, ligament, cartilage, and cardiovascular tissue.

Other molecules that hold fiber-forming collagens together include proteoglycans and calcium phosphate. Calcium phosphate linkages are similar to crosslinks. They increase modulus, decrease strain at failure, and increase UTS. At the molecular and fibrillar levels, calcium phosphate restricts collagen movement by binding to collagen sites. The presence of charge leads to bonds with charged amino acid R groups, whereas the presence of rigid ceramic plates inhibits more flexible collagen fibers.

3.3 ELASTIN

Elastin is a rubber-like protein in connective tissue, functioning as a "perfect coil." In terms of function, because it has coils in its structure, it allows tissues to resume their shape after stretching or contracting. Elastin is resistant to chemical and physical stresses and is not soluble in water, neutral salt solutions, dilute acid solutions, or dilute alkaline solutions at low temperatures. Elastin gives tissues the ability to reverse deformations, helping skin to return to its original position when it is poked or pinched, blood vessels to return to their normal size after expansion, and lungs to expand during breathing.

Elastin is found in blood vessels, with a higher concentration in aorta (Table 3.1),[8,9] as well as a high concentration in the lungs, and normal amounts in ligaments and tendons, skin, bladder, and elastic cartilage present in the outer ear, larynx, and epiglottis.

3.3.1 Elastin: Structure

The final three-dimensional structure of elastic fibers (elastin) and the fibers' interaction with other components of the ECM determine the mechanical properties of tissues. Elastin has a random coil conformation, which is composed of several randomly oriented coils (when relaxed). The coils, or spiral filaments, consist of peptide chains that can stretch out (Figure 3.14).[10] These chains are connected by specific amino acids (desmosin and isodesmosin). Elastin is mainly composed of glycine, valine, alanine, and proline. One third of the amino acids in elastin are glycine. This is similar to collagen and important for elastin's function. There are 830 amino acids in elastin, totaling up a molecular weight of 64 to 72 kDa. Glycine is distributed randomly throughout the elastin molecule, where in contrast, glycine is distributed evenly throughout the collagen

TABLE 3.1   Relative Concentrations of Elastin and Collagen in Various Tissues by Dry Weight

Tissue	Elastin (%)	Collagen (%)
Human skin	0.6–2.1	71.9
Human lung	3–7	10
Human aorta	28–32	12–24
Cow aorta	39.8	23.1
Pig aorta	57.1	16
Human Achilles tendon	4.4	86.0
Human liver	0.16–0.30	3.9
Cow liver	0	1.97
Pig liver	0	2.46

Source: Dermatology AAO, Dermatology curriculum: American academy of dermatology, Available from: http://www.aad.org/professionals/Residents/MedStudCoreCurr/DCElastin. htm, 2007; Neuman, R.E. and Logan, M.A., *J. Biol. Chem.*, 186, 549–556, 1950.

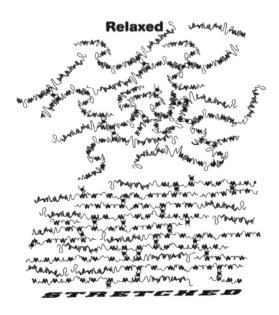

FIGURE 3.14 Drawing of elastin, randomly oriented when relaxed and aligned and ordered when stretched. (From Wang, M.C. et al., *Biomaterials*, 15, 507–512, 1994.)

molecule. The random distribution of glycine makes elastin hydrophobic. The inclusion of the glycine is important for elastin mechanical properties because the size of its side chain (just hydrogen) gives it more flexibility than the other amino acids in the molecule with larger side chains.

Elastin is formed when multiple tropoelastin molecules are covalently bonded together via crosslinks. Tropoelastin is the elastin precursor and is soluble. Tropoelastin is transported to the intercellular space by elastin-binding protein (EBP) and joins with microfibril proteins. Lysine residues in tropoelastin undergo oxidative deamination because of lysyl oxidase, forming desmosine- and isodesmosine-based crosslinks form. The crosslinking creates elastin but also decreases solubility, which is why elastic fibers are a highly insoluble in water. Elastin's hydrophobicity allows the molecules to slide over one another. This creates stretch and allows recoil in the tissue. The desmosine and isodesmosine crosslinks (covalent bonds) link four elastin molecules. Desmosine and isodesmosine are unique to elastin.

Tropoelastin contains both a-helix and beta sheet structures. Alanine and lysine rich segments lead to a-helices. Glycine-, proline-, and valine-rich segments lead to b-sheets. The a-helices form crosslinks because of lysine (allysine). Elastin is mainly found in the form of elastic fibers. Elastic fibers are composed of a large amorphous central core surrounded by a mesh of microfibrils. The core is composed of elastin, which gives elastic fibers a high capacity for stretch and recoil. Elastic fibers are formed through the deposit of tropoelastin onto a template of microfibrils, deposited by EBP. Microfibrils are composed of a mixture of several proteins including fibrillin. The microfibrils are oriented parallel to the direction of the applied force and are 10 nm wide, lying at the periphery of growing elastic fibers. Fibrillin is a glycoprotein that forms a sheath surrounding the amorphous elastin. Microfibrils are composed of end-to-end polymers of fibrillin.

3.3.2 Elastin: Assembly

Elastogenesis is a highly complex process that starts inside the cell. First the tropo-elastin molecule is synthesized. A 67-kDa galactolectin binds to it preventing it from aggregating intracellularly. This association lasts until the complex is excreted into the extracellular space. This process is guided by EBP. A companion chaperone interacts with galactosugars of the microfibrils. The microfibrillar component works as a scaffold for the deposition of elastin and may play a critical role in the correct alignment of the tropoelastin molecules. The interaction of the N-terminal part of the micro-fibrillar-associated glycoprotein with the C-terminal end of tropoelastin is required for normal elastogenesis. This is similar to collagen. Once aligned, most of the lysyl residues of the tropoelastin molecule are deaminated and oxidized to allysine. This requires lysyl oxidase. The crosslinks are then formed by the reaction of the allysines with themselves or with an unmodified lysine. This leads to the insolubilization of the tropoelastin chains as the elastin network grows.

Mature elastin is an insoluble polymer constituted by several or more tropoelastin molecules covalently bound to each other by crosslinks. These can be bi (lysinon-orleucine), tri(merodesmosine), or tetra-functional (desmosine and isodesmosine) in nature, and the increase in complexity is thought to progress as the fiber matures and ages. It starts by linking just two tropoelastin molecules together, then progresses to three and then four.

In between the rigid cross-linking domains, the hydrophobic segments exhibit a considerable mobility and contribute greatly to the entropy of the system. Despite its very hydrophobic nature, elastin is highly hydrated by both hydration water and solvent water that swells the polymer *in vivo*. Water enhances the entropy of the molecule.

The behavior of elastin is related to the presence of relevant amounts of glycine. This is a small amino acid that increases range of polypeptide motion. The glycine content has a positive correlation with the flexibility of the polypeptide chains. These protein elastomers are all characterized by anomalously high contents of glycine.

3.3.3 Elastin: Degradation

The body does not make elastin after the age of 12 or 13 (puberty). Once the body has made elastin, it will not make that protein any more, which means that damaged elastin will not be replaced. Over time, tissues lose their elasticity. Skin is a prime example.

Elastin can be damaged by smoking, stress, hormones, and UV light. Loss of elastin is considered a sign of aging. The loss of elastin decreases the efficiency of some organs and systems. Blood vessels lose their property to stretch easily. Damage to elastin in the trachea and lungs can cause breathing difficulties. Bladder function can become impaired. Over time, the sun's UV light damages the elastin in the skin, causing skin to lose its elasticity, forming wrinkles. Fragmented elastic fibers are hallmarks of sun-damaged skin.

3.3.4 Elastin: Arteries

Elastin is the principal ECM protein deposited by vascular smooth muscle cells in the arterial media. It contributes up to 50% of the vessel's dry weight. Elastin is secreted as a soluble monomer, tropoelastin. Following posttranslational modification, tropoelastin is cross-linked by lysyl oxidase and organized into elastin polymers that form concentric rings of elastic lamellae around the arterial lumen. Each elastic lamella alternates with a ring of smooth muscle forming a lamellar unit.

The role of elastin is not just structural; it controls artery aging and atherosclerosis and also acts as a barrier to solutes. Structural alterations to elastin are associated with repeated pulsations due to aging and heart rate. It has been shown that elastic lamellae grow increasingly fragmented and fibrotic with age, especially with hypertension, which proves bad for blood flow and vessel health. Elastin disruption occurs as atherosclerotic plaque progresses. Elastin is also involved in the trapping and retention of cholesterol in the intima. The early stages of atherosclerosis feature mainly low-density lipoproteins (LDL).

As an aside, some pharmaceuticals in clinical trials focus on elastin of blood vessels to stop the progression of atherosclerosis. The role of elastin as a barrier to solutes is related to its structure. Internal elastic lamina (IEL) is mainly composed of pure elastin coated with microfibrils. The IEL constitutes an otherwise impermeable barrier. There are pores in the IEL. The number of enlarged pores at arterial bifurcations increase in number with aging and increased blood flow. Simulations of the IEL have revealed that the shear stress surrounding a smooth muscle cell near a pore can be 100 times greater than that recorded away from the IEL.

The orientation of elastin in the aortic wall has elastic fibers of the internal elastic lamina parallel relative to luminal flow, whereas elastin fibers contained in elastic lamellae of media are perpendicular to blood flow. Elastic fibers in the media are oriented in a way that contains the circumferential mechanical stress of pulsation. The elastic fibers contained in internal elastic lamina can sustain longitudinal stress and act as a membrane. The arrangement of the elastic fibers is all about the circumferential and shear stress in the vessel.

The elastic lamellae are considered to be the functional and structural units of the arterial wall. Elastic lamellae provide the resilience to absorb the hemodynamic stress of cardiac systole and also release energy in the form of sustained blood pressure during diastole. In summary, elastin protects the vessel from stress overload through energy dissipation and propagates the pressure wave to move blood. It acts as a physical barrier, protecting the rest of the vessel.

An interesting note, the insoluble crosslinked elastin produced during late fetal and early postnatal development is stable with a slow turnover rate. It usually lasts for the entire life span of an organism. Elastin fibers may be degraded by numerous matrix metalloproteinases. They are present in latent forms under normal physiologic conditions and become activated following vessel wall injury.

3.3.5 Elastin: Diseased States

Elastin is responsible for the reversal of deformations in tissue. A decrease in elastin content or changes in elastin structure can result in pathological conditions, such as aneurysms or pulmonary emphysema. Diseased states that lead to genetic alterations in the amino acid sequence of elastin result in changes in tissue appearance and behavior. Supravalvular aortic stenosis (SVAS) is also known as Williams Syndrome (WS), a disease that causes significant narrowing of the large arteries and is inherited either as an isolated, autosomal dominant trait or as part of the WS. The WS is a rare genetic disorder characterized by mild to moderate mental retardation or learning difficulties. Those with WS have a distinctive facial appearance and a unique personality that combines overfriendliness and high levels of empathy with anxiety. WS is a developmental disorder involving the central nervous system and the connective tissues.

In SVAS, tropoelastin is truncated and thus lacks some cross-linking domains as well as the C-terminal region. This explains, in part, the deposition of abnormal elastic fibers. Because the elastic fibers are disorganized, SVAS may result from an adaptation of the vessels. These vessels are less elastic and subjected to persistent stress. This leads to smooth muscle hypertrophy and collagen deposition.

Cutis laxa is an elastin related disorder that causes the loss of elastin and elastic fibers in the cutaneous and other connective tissue layers. It can occur in both genetic and acquired forms. In a severe form, the elastic fibers are almost undetectable in the skin and internal organs. This leads to the early death of the patient. (Remember, elastin is important for lungs, arteries, etc.) Other cutis laxa phenotypes only lead to a mild wrinkling of the skin. The acquired form of cutis laxa is usually a consequence of loss of cutaneous elastic fibers because of local or generalized inflammation usually caused by increased elastolytic activity. Cutis laxa occurs as the crosslinks of elastin are incorrectly or not at all synthesized, leading to abnormal fibers. In some cases, there is a lack of the C-terminal region in tropoelastin. The abnormal tropoelastin molecules are unable to give the correct supramolecular structures.

Elastoderma is another disease whose symptoms look like cutis laxa (skin appearance). Elastoderma manifests itself with an elastin accumulation in the skin, where a large amount of elastic tissue is deposited throughout the dermis replacing the subcutaneous tissue. The ultrastructure of the elastic material differs significantly from that of normal elastin. Grape-like structures of elastin can be observed by scanning electron microscopy. These structures are similar to those observed when the polypeptide poly(VGVHypG) self-aggregates. Elastoderma could be a result of extensive hydroxylation of the prolyl residues of tropoelastin molecules. This creates the chaotic deposition of an elastin-like material.

3.4 PROTEOGLYCANS

Proteoglycans represent a special class of glycoproteins that are heavily glycosylated. They consist of a core protein with one or more covalently attached glycosaminoglycan chain(s); these molecules are charged and large. They serve a variety of purposes

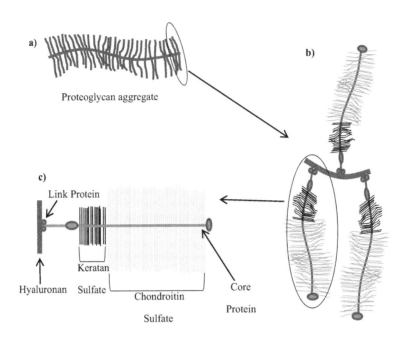

FIGURE 3.15   Drawing of the proteoglycan aggrecan, (a) in aggregate form, (b) a closer look at the aggregate, and (c) a detailed look at the proteoglycan structure.

in different tissues. Proteoglycans serve as shock absorbers; they bind cells to ECM. Proteoglycans keep water in the tissue, help organize collagen fibers, and play a role in wound healing (Figure 3.15).

Proteoglycans have a protein core connected to multiple glycosaminoglycan (GAG) chains that are covalently bonded to the protein core, Figure 3.15c. GAGs are long, unbranched polysaccharides consisting of a repeating disaccharide unit. The disaccharide unit consists of an N-acetyl-hexosamine and a hexose or hexuronic acid, either or both of which may be sulfated; hexoses include glucose, fructose, and galactose. Using a link protein several proteoglycans can bind together into larger structures (Figures 3.15a and b). The combination of the sulfate group and the carboxylate groups of the uronic acid residues gives them a very high density of negative charge. This helps them bring water to tissues. In cartilage, the large aggregating proteoglycans aggrecan and versican contribute 50% to 85% of the proteoglycans in the tissue. Small proteoglycans like biglycan and decorin contribute less than 10% of total proteoglycans.

Aggrecan has a size of $1-4 \times 10^6$ Da with a protein core of 220,000 to 250,000 Da, up to 50 keratan sulfate chains and 100 chondroitin sulfate chains attached. Aggrecan molecules can form macromolecular complexes of $300-400 \times 10^6$ Da. Aggrecan contributes to the mechanical and physicochemical properties of cartilage. Aggrecan monomers have two extended regions that carry the most of the GAGs and three globular domains, G1 and G2 at the N-terminus and G3 at the C-terminus of the core protein.

Aggrecan has a large amount of negatively charged polysaccharide chains (more than 10,000 negative charges). This creates an extremely high osmotic swelling pressure in cartilage. This swelling pressure is counteracted by the resistance of the intact collagen fibers in the matrix. This relationship between swelling pressure and physical resistance from the matrix provides cartilage with high compressive resistance and strength.

Biglycan is a nonaggregating proteoglycan. It has a molecular mass of approximately 100,000 Da with a protein core of 38,000 Da. Biglycan has two types of GAG chains, 40% to 50% are dermatan sulfate and the remainder are chondroitin sulfate. It is a member of the leucine-rich repeat (LRR) protein family.

Biglycan is important for ECM arrangement; it interacts with collagen VI. Conflicting data exists as to whether biglycan interacts with fibrillar collagens or not; it binds to collagen coatings but does not appear to precipitate with collagen fibers. Further studies show that biglycan organizes collagen VI assemblies into structured networks. This requires the intact molecule with its two glycosaminoglycan chains. Biglycan is also localized around cells. Biglycan bound to the N-terminal globular domain of collagen type VI at the same time can bind to matrilin-1, 2, or 3. The matrilin molecule can in turn reach the collagen molecules, collagen fibers as well as aggrecan.

Biglycan also interacts with transforming growth factor-β (TGF-β). TGF-β is a profibrotic key mediator in tissue fibrosis. TGF-β is one of the key profibrotic cytokines. It is chemotactic for fibroblasts, induces the synthesis of matrix proteins and glycoproteins, and inhibits collagen degradation by induction of protease inhibitors and reduction of metalloproteases. Biglycan has been shown to inhibit TGF-β *in vitro*. It has been suggested that biglycan (and other similar proteoglycans) may be able to sequester an overwhelming amount of TGF-β into the matrix and thereby control its biological effects.

Another small proteoglycan found in many collagenous tissues is decorin. It is a nonaggregating proteoglycan that is present in cartilage in molar amounts. It is the main proteoglycan in meniscus. It is also widely distributed in mesenchymal tissues, associated and bound to collagen. It interacts with fibrillar collagen using its core protein. Decorin binds at the d and e bands of collagen; this involves mainly the leucine-rich repeats of the core protein. Decorin binding influences collagen fibrillogenesis. The binding of decorin to fiber-forming collagens affects the collagen fibril diameter. A lack of decorin leads to thinner fibrils. Decorin knockout mice exhibit fragile skin, probably because of irregularly shaped collagen. Decorin folds on itself into a "U" shape and the arms of the "U" bind with two collagen molecules. This probably creates space between fibrils regulating fibril thickness.

Like biglycan, decorin also interacts with TGF-β. Decorin has been shown to inhibit TGF-β *in vitro* and *in vivo*. Decorin has been successfully employed to reduce tissue fibrosis in different disease models in kidney, lung, and vasculature.

There are some collagens that are also proteoglycans; these are called *FACIT collagens.* FACIT stands for fibril-associated collagens with interrupted triple helices. They are a family of collagens that don't form fibrils but are associated with the fibrillar collagens (types I and II). The FACIT share a common basic structure. They all have several triple helical domains (collagen type domains [Col]) separated by nontriple helical domains (NC). Data suggests that each of the FACIT collagens is glycosylated. FACIT collagens include Type IX, Type XII, Type XIV, and Type XIX (some data suggests this is also a FACIT collagen).

As stated previously, an important part of proteoglycans are the GAGs. GAGs vary in the type of hexosamine, hexose, or hexuronic acid unit they contain (e.g., glucuronic acid, iduronic acid, galactose, galactosamine, or glucosamine). One common GAG is chondroitin sulphate. It is a sulfated GAG composed of a chain of alternating sugars (N-acetylgalactosamine and glucuronic acid). Chondroitin sulfate A (Figure 3.16) is present in aggregating proteoglycans: aggrecan, versican, brevican, and neurocan. In aggrecan, *chondroitin sulfate A* is a major component of cartilage. The sulfate groups of chondroitin sulfate A generate electrostatic repulsion. Sulfates are tightly packed and highly charged; they provide much of the compression resistance in the tissue. A loss of chondroitin sulfate A from the cartilage is a major cause of osteoarthritis.

Dermatan sulfate or chondroitin sulfate B (Figure 3.17) is a GAG found mostly in skin, but also in blood vessels, heart valves, tendons, and lungs. Dermatan sulfate may have roles in coagulation, cardiovascular disease, carcinogenesis, infection, wound repair, and fibrosis. It is also referred to as *chondroitin sulfate B*.

Keratan sulfate (Figure 3.18) is a large, highly hydrated molecule that can act as a cushion in joints. It is also called *keratosulfate* and is found in the cornea,

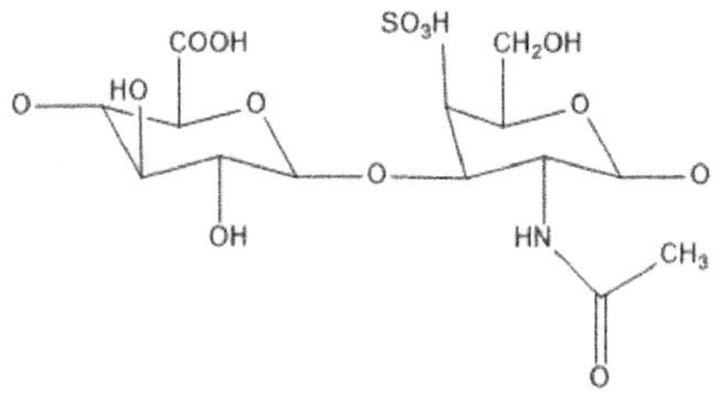

FIGURE 3.16 Chondroitin sulfate A.

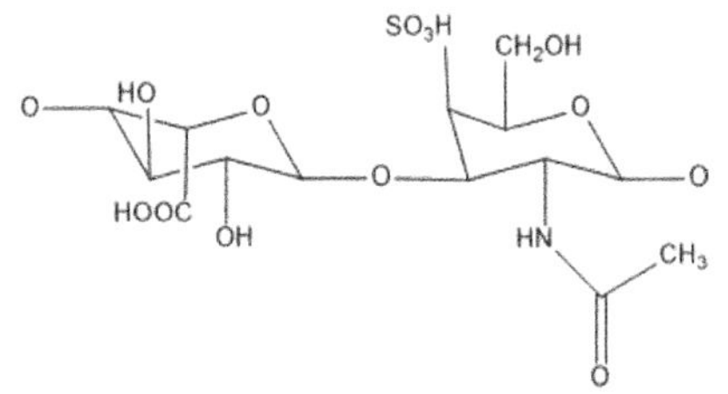

FIGURE 3.17 Dermatan sulfate (Chondroitin sulfate B).

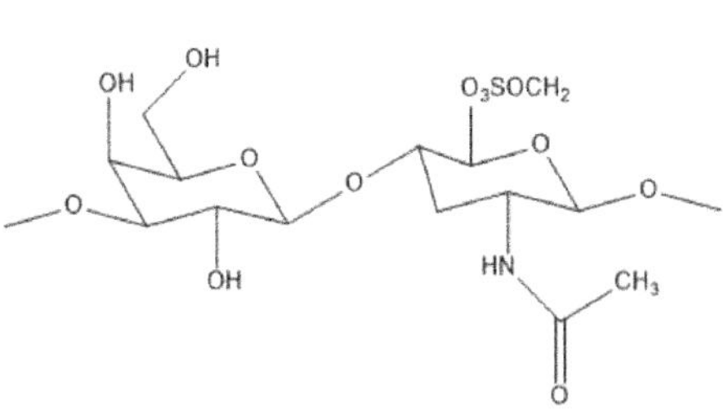

FIGURE 3.18 Keratan sulfate.

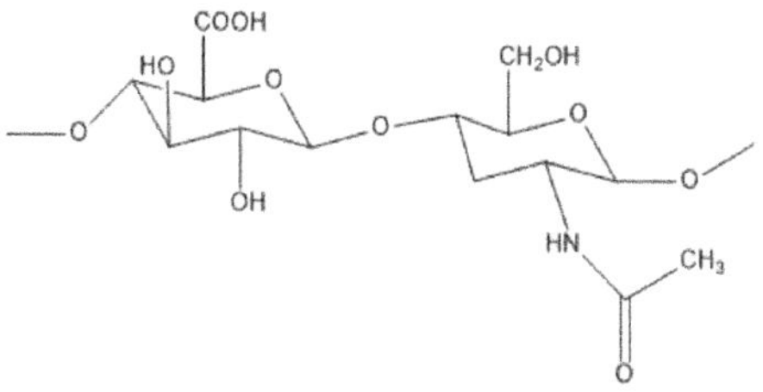

FIGURE 3.19   Heparan sulfate.

cartilage, and bone. Keratan sulfate is linked to tissue hydration in the cornea, which is important for the transparency of the tissue.

Heparin sulfate (Figure 3.19) is a linear polysaccharide found in all animal tissues. It binds to a variety of protein ligands. Heparin sulphate also regulates a wide variety of biological activities, including developmental processes, angiogenesis, and blood coagulation.

Heparin (Figure 3.20) is a highly sulfated GAG widely used as an injectable anticoagulant. It is also used to form an inner anticoagulant surface on various experimental and medical devices such as test tubes and renal dialysis machines. More recently it has been used in tissue engineering to improve cell proliferation (in small concentrations).

Hyaluronan (Figure 3.21) is a non-sulfated GAG that is found in many different tissues including connective tissue, epithelial tissue, and neural tissue. Hyaluronan contributes to cell proliferation and migration. Hyaluronan is a prominent component of articular cartilage, it coats chondrocytes. In cartilage aggrecan binds to hyaluronan in the presence of the link protein and forms large, highly negatively charged aggregates (Figure 3.15). These aggregates imbibe water and are responsible for the resilience of cartilage to compression. The molecular

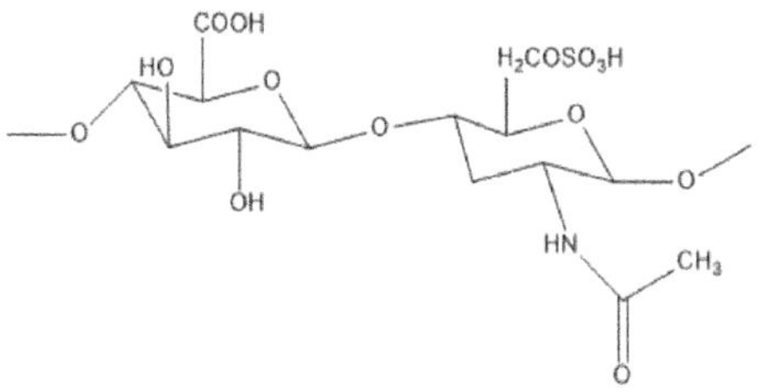

FIGURE 3.20   Heparin.

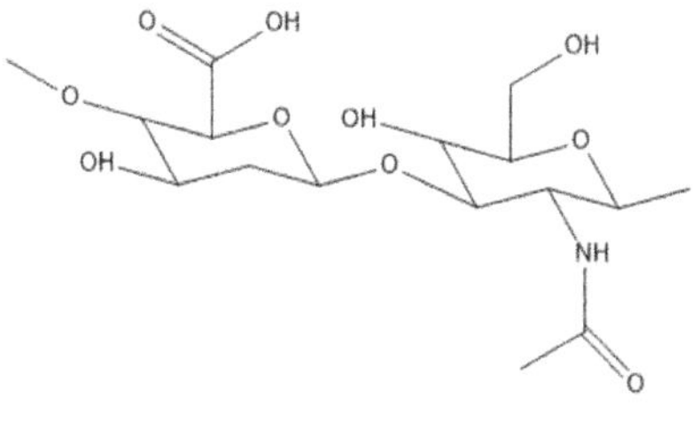

FIGURE 3.21   Hyaluronan.

weight of hyaluronan in cartilage decreases with age. Hyaluronan links the ECM with the chondrocytes. Chondrocytes have receptors on their surfaces that bind extracellular hyaluronan. It forms a direct linkage between the cells and the matrix. This matrix may provide an important mechanism by which chondrocytes can detect changes in the ECM. This linkage between the cells and matrix may play a role in cell-matrix mechanochemical transduction.

In articular cartilage there are molecular interactions between the proteoglycans and between the networks formed by collagens and the proteoglycan aggregates. These interactions can affect chondrocyte metabolism, collagen fibrillogenesis, and collagen network organization. The interactions existing between the collagen network and the proteoglycan aggregates are mainly a result of friction.

Proteoglycans do not contribute to the tensile stiffness and strength of the collagen network. The charge does alter mechanical properties indirectly through charge repulsion and hydration. There are molecular networks formed by proteoglycans in solution at physiological concentrations. These proteoglycan networks and the proteoglycan-collagen composite matrix formed *in vitro* are capable of storing elastic energy. Their shear stiffnesses are far lower than those for normal articular cartilage. These networks are responsible for compressive strength but not shear strength (directly). Proteoglycans are typically shear-thinning molecules; the viscosity of their solutions decreases with increases in the applied pressure.

The swelling pressure exerted by the fixed charge density of the proteoglycans serves to inflate the collagen network and helps to maintain the ECM organization. This inflated state also allows the collagen network to sustain tensile loads and thus provide shear stiffness to the ECM (indirectly).

Fibrillar collagen and proteoglycan synthesis are related in tissues. As noted, decorin has been found to bind to fibril-forming collagens and affects collagen fibrillogenesis *in vitro* and *in vivo*. Biglycan also plays a role in matrix organization though interactions with non-fibril–forming collagens that bind to fibril-forming collagens, among these non-fibril–forming collagens is collagen type VI. Aggrecan also aids in the organization of fibril formation. Studies have shown that decreases in aggrecan expression lead to abnormal collagen fibrils with increased diameter. Table 3.2 lists some common GAGs and their biological importance.

TABLE 3.2   List of Glycosaminoglycans: Their Location and Importance

GAG	Location	Importance
Hyaluronan	Synovial fluid, vitreous humor, ECM of loose connective tissue	Shock absorbing
Chondroitin sulfate	Cartilage, bone, heart valves	Most abundant, compression resistance
Heparan sulfate	Basement membranes, components of cell surfaces	Wound healing
Heparin	Component of intracellular granules of mast cells lining the arteries of the lungs, liver and skin	Wound healing
Dermatan sulfate	Skin, blood vessels, heart valves	Wound healing
Keratan sulphate	Cornea, bone, cartilage aggregated with chondroitin sulfates	Cushion in joints

3.5 BIOLOGICAL MINERAL (CALCIUM PHOSPHATE)

Calcium phosphate makes up a majority of the mineral present in bone. Hydroxyapatite (HAP), $Ca_{10}(PO_4)_6(OH)_2$, is the predominant calcium phosphate in mature bone. Hydroxyapatite crystallizes in a hexagonal crystal system. Tissues mineralize under a variety of conditions. Some mineralize as a part of normal development, whereas others mineralize when in a diseased state. Bones and turkey gastrocnemius tendons are examples of tissues that normally mineralize. This usually takes place in tissues that require increased stiffness and load-bearing capability. Examples of diseased state mineralization include: calciphylaxis, dermatomyositis, calcergy, and steogenesis imperfecta.

3.5.1 Biological Mineral: The Mineralization Process

There are other types of calcium phosphate in bone, not just HAP, although it is the main type. Other types of calcium phosphate present include amorphous calcium phosphate, tricalcium phosphate, brushite, and octacalcium phosphate. There are different theories about the formation of mineral, specifically HAP in bone. It is theorized that amorphous calcium phosphate is composed of mainly tricalcium phosphate. The Ca^{2+} and PO_4 ions begin to aggregate in a simple manner and then over time form a more complex, crystalline structure[11,12] (Figure 3.22). As time passes, the amorphous material would be converted into a crystalline mineral. This process would be hindered by the presence of inhibitors such as adenosine triphosphate (ATP), pyrophosphate, diphosphate, and some phospholipids. Another theory suggests that other types of calcium phosphate are produced as precursors, which are then hydrolyzed into HAP. It has been proposed that other calcium phosphates (such as octacalcium phosphate or brushite) are initially produced and then converted into

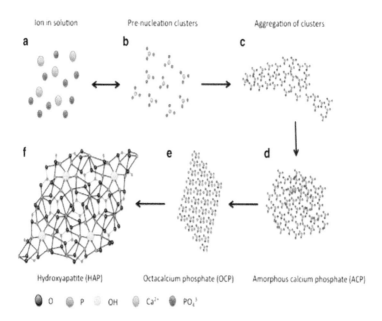

FIGURE 3.22 The steps of hydroxyapatite formation. (From Cai, M.M. et al. *BoneKEy Re.*, 4, 672, 2015; Habraken, W.J. et al., *Nat. Commun.*, 4, 1507, 2013.)

HAP (Figure 3.22). Tricalcium phosphate, $Ca_3(PO_4)_2$, (also known as calcium orthophosphate, tertiary calcium phosphate, and tribasic calcium phosphate) is one of the main combustion products of bone (bone ash). Another common form of calcium phosphate is brushite (also known as Dicalcium Phosphate Dihydrate [DCPD]). It is a hydrated calcium phosphate with the composition $CaHPO_4 \cdot 2H_2O$. It is usually the calcium phosphate source of kidney stones.

Octacalcium phosphate, $Ca_8H_2(PO_4)_6 5H_2O$, has a layered structure involving apatitic and hydrated layers. Apatitic layers have calcium and phosphate distributed in a manner similar to that for HAP. Hydrated layers contain lattice water and less densely packed calcium and phosphate ions. Hydrated layer may form an interphase between HAP and the surrounding solution. These apatites have lower surface tensions and free energy barriers for nucleation, which means less energy is required to form them compared to HAP. They are less complex and could serve as crystalline intermediates to HAP.

The mitochondria may play a role in mineralization. It is known that the mitochondria in different tissues store Ca_2. When $CaPO_4$ is stored in the mitochondria it is usually in the form of amorphous calcium phosphate. This is especially true in the mitochondria of cells in tissues that are being mineralized. This presents the possibility that this amorphous calcium phosphate may be released during mineralization. It is hypothesized that this amorphous calcium phosphate is mainly composed of tricalcium phosphate; leading to the previous theory that the Ca_2 and PO_4 ions could aggregate in a simple manner and then over time form a more complex, crystalline structure.

3.5.2 Biological Mineral: Nucleation

The biological nucleation of calcium phosphate is dependent on several parameters, the concentrations of calcium and phosphate ions in solution, the presence of collagen, and the presence of various other macromolecules. For mineralization to occur there has to be a readily available source of calcium and phosphate ions to propagate crystal growth. Some *in vitro* studies accomplish this by supersaturated solutions in order to promote apatite crystal precipitation. This can be done with mineralizing media and concentrated simulated body fluid (SBF). *In vivo*, fluids such as blood and extracellular fluid do not have high enough concentrations of calcium and phosphate ions to cause spontaneous precipitation of apatite crystals at physiological pH. However, the concentrations are high enough to support crystal nucleation once it begins. An example of this can be seen in a study on cartilage matrix fluid, by Howell in 1968, where the investigators aspirated fluid from the area of initial calcification in growth plate cartilage.[13,14] It was found that the calcium and phosphate concentrations were too low to begin apatite precipitation (1.6 and 2.0 mM, respectively, at a pH of 7.53). On the other hand, these concentrations could support crystal growth if a few nucleating crystals of hydroxyapatite were present (Figure 3.23).

Collagen has long been recognized as an initiator of mineralization that promotes apatite crystal growth. Studies have also shown that type I collagen also serves as a guide for crystal proliferation. During mineralization calcium phosphate crystals align with the collagen long axis.[5,15] Studies of mineralization of self-assembled collagen fibrils and in turkey tendons suggest that mineralization begins in the gap region and then subsequently spreads to the overlap region.[5] Crystal nucleation occurs first in the gap region, then spreads onto overlap region of

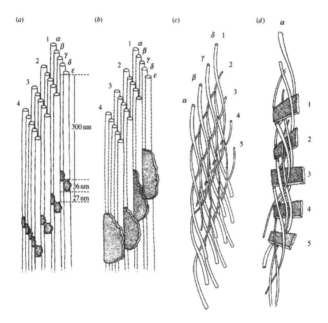

FIGURE 3.23   Models of collagen mineralization based on early collagen models and more recent models. (Taken from Alexander, B. et al., *Interface*, 9, 1774–1786, 2012.)

type I collagen. The gaps are three dimensional, and the nucleation eventually spreads throughout the fibril and fiber. The crystals develop lengthwise along the collagen long axes, eventually forming sheets of mineral parallel to each other along the long axis of the collagen fibers.[5,15] The alignment of crystals increases mechanical properties. Landis argues that the quarter-staggered arrangement of the collagen molecules creates grooves and channels in the fibrils.[5] These areas promote ordered crystal growth along the collagen long axis by lowering the local concentration of ions. These grooves and channels are the result of collagen self-assembly. This process requires precise alignment of neighboring molecules and the presence of gap and overlap regions that run continuously across fibers. Traub, et al. have identified the area around the e band in the gap region as the first nucleation site.[16] This data agrees with a previous study that links the presence of mineral during early stages of mineralization with less hydrophobic areas in the collagen molecule. The least hydrophobic areas have the most charges, which can attract calcium and phosphate ions and lead to mineral nucleation. This area (the e band) is the least hydrophobic area of the gap region. The gap region is less hydrophobic than the overlap region. This makes the e band in the gap region more likely to be an area of early nucleation site. The gap region creates three-dimensional grooves throughout tissue, possibly an area of increased local ion concentration. These are places for mineral growth to occur throughout a fiber.

3.5.3 Biological Mineral: Other Molecules

Various macromolecules *in vivo* are important to mineralization. They can promote or prevent nucleation in a number of ways. Phosphoproteins have been identified in dentin and calcified cartilage. They are believed to play a role in apatite nucleation. The arrangement of the phosphate groups in these proteins can be used to bind calcium and providing sites for apatite nucleation.[17] Proteoglycans are found in the matrices of both calcifying and noncalcifying tissues and are composed of GAG chains and a protein core. Various proteoglycans such as bovine nasal proteoglycan have been shown to slow the conversion of amorphous calcium phosphate into phosphate and the nucleation of HAP from calcium and phosphate ions. The GAGs in these macromolecules are highly charged, which gives them a strong affinity for calcium and may bind to calcium in solution and also prevents calcium from forming apatite crystals. Therefore, the removal of proteoglycans from the extracellular matrix may promote mineralization. Phospholipids are found in human bone and the mineralization front of articular cartilage. Acidic phospholipids have a strong affinity for ionic calcium. These molecules induce apatite formation *in vitro* by acting as calcium traps at the site of nucleation. They form complexes with calcium that are believed to have structural features that promote apatite nucleation.

3.5.4 Biological Mineral: Strain

Other studies have also shown a link between physical strain (a change in length) in tissues and mineralization. Work by Ascenzi shows a possible link between strain in tissues and mineralization.[18] In both studies, lamellae separated from osteons shrink when cut, which demonstrates the presence of initial strain before mineralization. A study on chick embryo tibias performed by Amprino[19] also shows that strain may be necessary for mineralization. Amprino inverted the tibial portions of chick embryos to reduce stress in that section during development, which led to poor development, including delayed ossification.

Mineral may also bind to charged residues on collagen fibers. Studies have shown that stretching collagen fibers after formation *in vitro* causes a decrease in swelling ratio (diameter before hydration divided by diameter after hydration) with an increase in strain.[20] In these studies, strain caused an increase in UTS. Stretching the fiber caused the fibrils to axially align and pack closer together because of the lateral contraction of the fibers. These interactions may have been induced by the charged residues of the amino acids on the surfaces of the fibrils. Strain and charged areas may lead to nucleation of mineral. Other studies have shown an increase in calcium phosphate deposition on reconstituted collagen fibers with an increase in strain before mineralization. Straining the fiber may expose charged areas in some of the flexible regions of the collagen molecules. The exposed charged areas could act as nucleation sites for calcium phosphate.[20]

3.5.5 Biological Mineral: Diseased States

Many diseases result in abnormal deposition of hydroxyapatite crystals in tissues. Notable ones include calciphylaxis, dermatomyositis, calcergy, and osteogenesis imperfecta. In all of these cases, although the mineral is deposited in different forms, the condition is a result of faulty collagen that leads to abnormally shaped HAP crystals. Calciphylaxis is characterized by a loose organization of collagen fibrils and extrafibrilar mineralization. The mineral forms a cylinder around the individual fibrils, where there is very little interfibrilar mineralization. The mineral is closely associated to one fibril.

Dermatomyositis is characterized by the presence of numerous collagen fibrils being laid down in a disorganized manner. Hydroxyapatite crystals associate with individual fibers, where the crystals are short, thin spears that are not oriented with the collagen long axis. There is little evidence of intercrystal association.

Calcergy is characterized by the presence of widely separated collagen bundles. Mineralization begins within the fibrils, where the HAP grows down the fibril and then grows radially. Early crystals are long, solid rods with tapered ends.

Osteogenesis imperfecta is caused by an overhydroxylation of the lysine residues because of the impeded nature of the collagen triple helix. The collagen fibrils are twisted or kinked and are not arranged in the 64–67-nm period. They have a smaller diameter and elastic modulus than normal collagen. The crystals in this diseased state form spikes that are not aligned along the collagen long axis. Lack of alignment and crystal continuity leads to a decrease in mechanical properties and possible voids in crystal matrix. The common theme of these diseases is that problems with collagen lead to problems with mineral.

3.5.6 Biological Mineral: Properties

Mineralization of a collagenous tissue results in stiffening of the tissue, creating an increased UTS, lower strain to failure, and an increased elastic modulus. Tissues can resist more force but are less ductile, which makes them more brittle. This is good for tissues such as bone and turkey tendon. The increase in strength creates a decrease in flexibility, which is bad for heart valves and blood vessels that need more flexibility. The mechanical behavior of bone has been shown to be related to the distribution, volume fraction, and amount of interphasic bonding of the mineral in the organic matrix. In conclusion, mechanical properties are linked to the amount of mineral, mineral continuity, where it is placed, and bonding between mineral and collagen. When there is a problem with one of these steps, things can go very wrong. Biological mineral also has the ability to bind to macromolecules directly. Binding is a result of charge-charge interactions. When used in tissue-engineered scaffolds, the negative phosphate groups present in calcium phosphate such as HAP increases the number of negative charges. This increases its ionic-binding potential and can be used to bind groups to enhance bone regeneration. This strategy is also used to inactivate groups, create a reservoir of chemical species, lead sustained release for prolonged effect, and lead to a burst release for a sudden effect. The binding of different species can also affect mineral metabolism, which is important for calcium balance. Chemical compounds that bind to HAP include salivary proteins, polyphosphates, amino acids, complement factors, polycarboxylamines, phosphate esters, and antibiotics. This is used by stains such as AlizarinRed. This strategy can be exploited by certain drugs that target bone and teeth. Biphosphonates have been investigated for these purposes.

QUESTIONS

1. What are proteins composed of?

2. What are the differences among the primary, secondary, tertiary, and quaternary structures of a protein

3. What amino acid repeat is necessary for collagen tripple helical structure?

4. Name two ways to increase the strength of collagen?

5. Name two tasks for elastin in blood vessels.

6. How do proteoglycans alter tissue stiffness?

7. How does mineralization affect tissue mechanical properties?

8. What is the major type of mineral in bone? In what form is the majority of it found?

9. Diseased mineralization states are typically caused by problems with which molecule?

10. Name different ways to increase the strength of a collagenous matrix.

REFERENCES

1. Silver FH, Freeman JW et al. Collagen self-assembly and the development of tendon mechanical properties. *Journal of Biomechanics.* 2003 36(10):1529–1553.
2. Pins GD, Christiansen DL et al. Self-assembly of collagen fibers. Influence of fibrillar alignment and decorin on mechanical properties. *Biophysical Journal.* 1997 73(4):2164–2172.
3. Wang MC, Pins GD et al. Collagen fibres with improved strength for the repair of soft tissue injuries. *Biomaterials.* 1994 15(7):507–512.
4. Silver FH, Freeman JW et al. Molecular basis for elastic energy storage in mineralized tendon. *Biomacromolecules.* 2001 2(3):750–756.
5. Landis WJ, Song MJ et al. Mineral and organic matrix interaction in normally calcifying tendon visualized in three dimensions by high-voltage electron microscopic tomography and graphic image reconstruction. *Journal of Structural Biology.* 1993 110(1):39–54.
6. McAllion SJ, Paterson CR. Causes of death in osteogenesis imperfecta. *Journal of Clinical Pathology.* 1996 49(8):627–630.
7. Paterson CR, Ogston SA et al. Life expectancy in osteogenesis imperfecta. BMJ. 1996 312(7027):351.
8. Dermatology AAo. Dermatology curriculum: American academy of dermatology; 2007. Available from: http://www.aad.org/professionals/Residents/MedStudCoreCurr/DCElastin.htm.
9. Neuman RE, Logan MA. The determination of collagen and elastin in tissues. *The Journal of Biological Chemistry.* 1950 186(2):549–556.
10. Gacko M. Elastin: Structure, properties and metabolism. *Cell and Molecular Biology Letters.* 2000 5(3):327–348.
11. Habraken WJ, Tao J et al. Ion-association complexes unite classical and non-classical theories for the biomimetic nucleation of calcium phosphate. *Nature Communications.* 2013 4:1507.
12. Cai MM, Smith ER et al. The role of fetuin-A in mineral trafficking and deposition. *BoneKEy Reports.* 2015 4:672.
13. Howell DS, Carlson L. Alterations in the composition of growth cartilage septa during calcification studied by microscopic x-ray elemental analysis. *Experimental Cell Research.* 1968 51(1):185–195.
14. Howell DS, Pita JC et al. Partition of calcium, phosphate, and protein in the fluid phase aspirated at calcifying sites in epiphyseal cartilage. *Journal of Clinical Investigation.* 1968 47(5):1121–1132.
15. Alexander B, Daulton TL et al. The nanometre-scale physiology of bone: Steric modelling and scanning transmission electron microscopy of collagen–mineral structure. *Interface.* 2012 9(73):1774–1786.
16. Traub W, Arad T et al. Origin of mineral crystal growth in collagen fibrils. *Matrix.* 1992 12(4):251–255.
17. Lee SL, Veis A et al. Dentin phosphoprotein: An extracellular calcium-binding protein. *Biochemistry.* 1977 28 16(13):2971–2979.
18. Ascenzi MG. A first estimation of prestress in so-called circularly fibered osteonic lamellae. *Journal of Biomechanics.* 1999 32(9):935–942.
19. Amprino R. The influence of stress and strain in the early development of shaft bones: An experimental study on the chick embryo tibia. *Anatomy and Embryology.* 1985 172(1):49–60.
20. Freeman JW, Silver FH. The effects of prestrain and collagen fibril alignment on in vitro mineralization of self-assembled collagen fibers. *Connective Tissue Research.* 2005 46(2):107–115.

CHAPTER 4

Tissue Structure and Function

4.1 INTRODUCTION

Before we can regenerate or "engineer" a tissue, we must first investigate the tissue. What are its functions, what is it made up of? What is its underlying architecture? In this section we will discuss the tissues of the body and how the structure of these tissues leads to their function in the body. As in most of the sections in this book, we will provide an overview of some important points with regard to each tissue. For more in-depth information we encourage you to seek other texts including the ones that we used for our background research. These texts include *Physiology*, edited by Berne, Levy, Koeppen, and Stanton; *Vander's Human Physiology: The Mechanisms of Body Function*, edited by Widmaier, Raff, and Strang; *Basic Orthopaedic Biomechanics*, edited by Mow and Hayes; *Human Physiology*, edited by Roades and Pflanzer; and *Tissue Mechanics* by Cowin and Doty.[1–5]

We will start with the most basic question: What is a tissue? A tissue is a group of cells with similar function and appearance. Specifically, a biological tissue is a collection of interconnected cells that perform a similar function within an organism. In our bodies, different organs have different functions, so they need different tissues to work together to carry out these functions. Although some tissues differ in their compositions, we find that many tissues are composed of the same large molecules. The differences lie in the amounts of these molecules and their arrangement in each tissue. Biological tissues vary in their thickness and complexity. The simplest tissues are found as membranes or sheets. These tissues combine to form organs, groups of organs form a system, and multiple systems make up the human body.

4.2 TYPES OF TISSUES

There are four basic types of tissues in the body, and each has a different function and different properties depending on the function. The four major types of tissues are connective, epithelial, muscular, and nervous. These tissues compose all of the organs and structures in the body.

Epithelial tissue covers the body surface and forms the lining for most internal cavities. The major function of epithelial tissue is protection, secretion, absorption, and filtration. Epithelial tissues are composed of layers of cells that cover organ surfaces. Examples include the surface of the skin and the inner lining of the digestive tract. The skin is an organ that is made up of epithelial tissue. It protects the body from dirt, dust, bacteria, microbes, and heat. Cells of the epithelial tissue have different shapes depending on the layer they are in. Shapes include thin and flat, cubic, or elongated.

Connective tissue is the most abundant tissue in the body and is the most widely distributed tissue type. Connective tissues have a variety of forms and functions. They serve as mechanical support and injury protection, or basically, tissue that holds everything together. Some people consider blood a connective tissue. Other connective tissues include fat tissue, dense fibrous tissue, cartilage, bone, and lymph. Extensive extracellular matrix (ECM) is an often used example. It is found in bones, ligaments and tendons, and cartilage.

Nervous tissue composes the central nervous system, brain, spinal cord, and peripheral nervous system. This tissue is responsible for the conversion of stimuli into electrical signals, the transfer of electrical signals, the processing of signals, and the stimulation of tissues and organs as a result of processed signals.

In muscle tissue, muscle cells contain contractile filaments that move past each other and change the size of the cell. There are three types of muscle. Smooth muscle is found in the inner linings of organs. Skeletal muscle is attached to bone, and cardiac muscle is found in the heart. Skeletal muscle is a voluntary type of muscle used in limb movement and locomotion. Smooth muscle is an involuntary type of muscle found in the walls of internal organs and blood vessels. Cardiac muscle is found only in the heart walls and is an involuntary type of muscle.

The properties of these tissues are governed by their biomacromolecules. The chemistry of these molecules leads to their strength and other properties (hydrophobic, hydrophilic, attractions to other molecules, ability to bind with other molecules, conductivity, etc.).

The arrangement of these molecules gives the tissue their mechanical properties. Fiber-forming biomacromolecules such as collagens can be arranged in several ways to give tissues unique mechanical properties. One arrangement is a random orientation. In this arrangement, the fibers are not well organized. This gives the tissue uniform strength in all directions. This type of arrangement can be seen in skin or facia. Fiber-forming biomacromolecules can also be aligned in one major direction. This gives the tissue enhanced strength in that direction, this is seen in tendon. Tissues can also have fiber-forming biomacromolecules that are aligned along multiple axes or alignable. The organization of these tissues becomes more aligned along one major axis when stress is applied.

Biological tissues range in thickness and complexity. The simplest are membranes or sheets and combine to form organs, which then combine to form a system. All of these tissues are complex, and organization begins at the molecular level and continues to the macro level. The organization of the collagen fibers in ligaments and tendons lead to enhanced mechanical properties. The arrangement of myofibers allows for the proper function of muscle. There are multiple layers, each with a different architecture. The cortical and trabecular bone each give bone strength under different loading conditions. In the skin, each layer serves a different functional purpose, from mechanical strength to warmth, etc.

Tissues are composed of proteins, proteoglycans, water, cells, and minerals. Structural proteins provide the shape and mechanical properties of the tissue. The chemistry of the proteins determine their strength and hence, tissue strength. The following molecular characteristics affect molecule and tissue properties. Molecular length determines tissue properties. Longer molecules can make more interactions with nearby molecules because of the available space on the molecule. This could lead to more chemical bonds or entanglements forming with like molecules, increasing tissue strength. The charge of the molecule is also of great importance. Charge-charge interactions can affect tissue strength through repulsion with like molecules or attracting water. This effect becomes magnified if the charged molecules are also large. For proteins, the nature of the side groups is important. Their size and chemistry determine how the protein folds into its three-dimensional structure, and therefore how it interacts with neighboring molecules. It can present charged areas for interactions with other charged molecules, it could allow for water-mediated bonds, etc. Two of the biomacromolecules that we will discuss in more detail are proteins and proteoglycans.

Proteins are long polymer chains of amino acids. Amino acids combine to form peptide units (polypeptides), which combine to form proteins. Proteins have a variety of different functions in the body. Among these functions are serving as structural materials in the ECM, and they make up enzymes and cell surface markers. Proteoglycans are long, highly charged molecules. Their charge attracts water into the tissue, and in some cases, they use charge repulsion to increase tissue mechanical properties and to prevent catastrophic tissue failure. Water itself is necessary for cell growth, and the removal of water during strain (tensile or compressive) is important for tissue mechanical properties. Biological minerals include calcium phosphate, which increases tissue stiffness and is stored in the calcium reservoirs of the body.

Tissue organization begins at the molecular level and continues to the macro level. The organization of the molecules in these tissues, primarily the proteins, impacts the behavior of the tissues. In ligaments and tendons, the primary structural protein, type I collagen, is arranged in a way that is primarily aligned with the tissue long axis. This leads to enhanced tissue strength in that direction. In skeletal muscle, cells fuse and arrange their contractile proteins so that they align, allowing the muscle to contract uniformly. In the next section, we will look at tissues from each of the categories and describe their architecture and discuss how this relates to the function of each tissue.

4.3 BLOOD VESSELS

As mammals, we have a closed blood vascular system. Blood is transported from the heart to all different parts of the body and back through a set of closed tubes. To transport blood efficiently, our bodies use different types of vessels.

To perform their specific tasks, human blood vessels differ in structure and function. There are three major types of blood vessels: arteries, veins, and capillaries. They each have

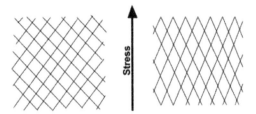

FIGURE 4.1 Schematic of an alignable network. The fibers in the material align in the direction of the applied stress.

different functions, structures, and properties. Blood leaves the heart through the arteries, which are elastic vessels that conduct the oxygenated blood (except in the case of the pulmonary artery) to the various tissues and organs. Deoxygenated blood returns from the tissues and organs to the heart via veins (except the pulmonary vein). The exchange of oxygen, carbon dioxide, nutrients, and waste between the blood and the tissue fluid occur in capillaries.

These larger blood vessels are examples of alignable collagen networks (Figure 4.1) with elastic tissue networks. They are alignable because the collagen fibers in these tissues become aligned with the direction of the largest stress created by the blood flowing through them. This direction is circumferential to the vessel.

4.3.1 Arteries

Arteries are elastic vessels. They dampen the pulsatile flow of blood from the heart, providing a more continuous flow to the tissues. The largest artery of the body is the aorta; it originates from the heart and branches out into smaller arteries called *arterioles*, which branch into capillaries. Arterioles are a major site of resistance to blood flow and are major determinants of blood flow in a tissue bed and distribution of blood to different tissue beds.

The muscular wall of the artery helps the heart pump blood. When the heart beats, the artery expands as it fills with blood. Arterial pressure varies between the peak pressure during heart contraction (systolic pressure) and the minimum (diastolic pressure) between contractions. When the heart relaxes, the artery contracts and exerts a force that is strong enough to push the blood along. This rhythm between the heart and the artery increases circulatory efficiency. Your pulse is the expansion and contraction of an artery. The arteries keep pace with heart contractions and therefore, can be used to measure heart rate.

Arteries (and veins) have three layers: the adventitia, the media, and the intima (Figure 4.2). The adventitia is the strong outermost layer and contains fibroblasts, large-diameter collagen fibrils, elastic fibers, and proteoglycans. It connects the arteries to surrounding tissues and prevents the vessel from tearing under pressure. The fibers allow the arteries to stretch and prevent overexpansion because of the pressure caused by blood flow.

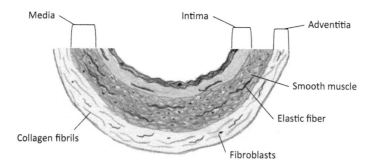

FIGURE 4.2 Arterial cross-section. The drawing shows all three layers, intima, media, and adventitia.

The media is the middle layer and also the muscular layer. It is composed of smooth muscle, collagen, and elastic fibers, whose presence makes this layer responsible for the bulk of the mechanical properties. Arterial mechanical properties are affected by the structure and thickness of the media. In the aorta, the media is about 550 micrometers thick (made of 50–65 layers). The smooth muscle cells are surrounded by a basement membrane, attached to dermatan sulfate, and associated with collagen fibrils. The collagen in the media is mainly type I and III and is distributed throughout the media as large-diameter wavy fibrils that are attached to dermatan sulfate with hyaluronic acid.

In the media, the collagen fibers are woven between layers of elastic fibers and smooth muscle cells, arranging them in parallel mechanically. They are all arranged in concentric rings called *elastic lamellae*, which wrap around the lumen (Figure 4.3). The collagen content changes in different arteries and is higher in the thoracic aorta than the abdominal aorta. The collagen prevents total failure of the tissue.

Elastic fibers have an amorphous elastin core with a rim of microfibrillar protein. Elastin makes up to 50% of the vessel's dry weight. Elastic fibers are organized into concentric rings of elastic lamellae around the arterial lumen. Each elastic lamella alternates with a ring of smooth muscle, forming a lamellar unit. The elastic lamellae are considered to be the functional and structural unit of the arterial wall; it provides the resilience to absorb

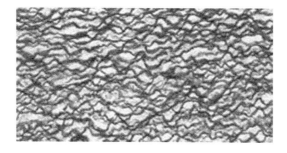

FIGURE 4.3 Stained elastic lamellae, dark fibers are elastin. (From https://basicmedicalkey.com/smooth-muscle-and-the-cardiovascular-and-lymphatic-systems/.)

the hemodynamic stress of cardiac systole. Structural alterations to elastin are linked to repeated pulsations because of aging and heart rate. Elastic lamellae become increasingly fragmented and damaged with age, especially with hypertension. Elastic fibers and collagen fibers in the media are oriented in a way that contains the circumferential mechanical stress of pulsation (Figure 4.3). The arrangement also allows for the release of energy in the form of sustained blood pressure during diastole.

The intima is the inner layer of arteries that contains epithelial cells and is comprised of an elastic membrane lining and smooth endothelium that is covered by elastic tissue. Here the elastin also controls artery aging, atherosclerosis, and acts as a barrier to solutes. The hollow internal cavity in which the blood flows is called the *lumen*.

Elastin is also involved in the trapping and retention of cholesterol in the intima during the early stages of atherosclerosis, caused by low-density lipoproteins (LDL). The growth of atherosclerotic plaque causes elastin damage in the intima. Elastin here acts as a barrier to solutes. The elastic fibers contained in internal elastic lamina (IEL) can sustain longitudinal stress. IEL is mainly composed of pure elastin coated with microfibrils and constitutes an otherwise impermeable barrier.

So the orientation of elastin in artery depends on the layer that it is in. Elastic fibers of the internal elastic lamina are parallel relative to luminal flow, whereas elastin fibers contained in elastic lamellae of media are perpendicular to blood flow. The orientation is the same for collagen fibers.

After arteries reach different tissue beds, they divide into smaller arterioles. The diameter of an arteriole is much smaller than an artery and is an important factor in blood flow resistance. Resistance is equal to a/r^4, so cutting the diameter in half raises the resistance by a factor of 16! Arterioles can dynamically change diameter due to arrangement of smooth muscle around the vessels (Figure 4.4). Contraction of smooth muscle decreases diameter and increases resistance. Arterioles have relatively more smooth muscle than other blood vessels in the body, and therefore resistance to blood flow through a tissue is almost entirely determined by the arterioles.

4.3.2 Veins

The veins contain a major portion of the circulating blood volume. At any one time approximately 75% of the blood is in the veins, which provide a conduit for the return of blood to the heart. The veins also regulate the distribution of blood volume in the body. The return

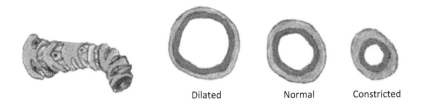

Dilated   Normal   Constricted

FIGURE 4.4 Drawing of smooth muscle surrounding an arteriole from the outside and cross-sections when dilated, normal, and constricted, based on figure by Berne, Levy, and Koeppen[1].

of blood to the heart is facilitated by large-diameter veins, one-way venous valves, skeletal muscle contraction, and respiration.

Veins are elastic vessels that transport deoxygenated blood from tissues to the heart, ranging in size from 1 millimeter to 11.5 centimeters in diameter. Venules are the smallest veins in the body. They receive blood from the arteries via the arterioles and capillaries. The venules branch into larger veins, which eventually carry the blood to the largest vein in the body, the vena cava. The blood is then transported from the vena cava to the right atrium of the heart.

To facilitate blood flow from venules to the heart, the body has large-diameter veins. Remember resistance to flow is proportional to radius,[4] so a large radius gives you less resistance. This is necessary because there is only a 10 mm Hg pressure drop between venules and the heart (right atrium), meaning that there is not a large amount of pressure pushing the blood to the heart. Like arteries, veins also have three layers: the adventitia, media, and intima (Figure 4.5).

The adventitia is the strong outer covering of veins, composed of connective tissue, collagen, and elastic fibers. These fibers allow the veins to stretch to prevent overexpansion because of the pressure that is exerted on the walls by blood flow. The media is the middle layer of the walls of veins and is composed of smooth muscle and elastic fibers. This layer is not as thick in veins as it is in arteries and does not pump very actively in veins. Blood in the veins is moved through the contraction of surrounding muscles on to the veins.

This is why blood can collect in your legs if you stand for long periods of time, such as soldiers at attention. This also happens when you sit for long periods of time such as on plane trips. To maintain blood flow you must be active, so when standing for long periods of time you should contract the muscles in your thighs, forcing blood to travel up, back to the heart. On planes you should get up and walk around the cabin.

The inner layer of the veins is also called the *intima*; this intima does not contain the elastic membrane lining that is found in arteries. The intima layers in some veins contain valves (Figure 4.5). The hollow internal cavity in which the blood flows is called the *lumen*. Valves prevent the back flow of blood and are necessary because there is little or no active pumping in veins. Back flow is prevented, and blood is pumped up from each section using muscle contraction.

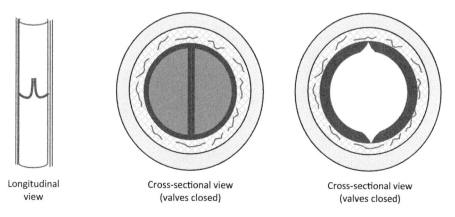

Longitudinal view   Cross-sectional view (valves closed)   Cross-sectional view (valves closed)

FIGURE 4.5   Views of a vein showing the valves and different layers, adventitia, media, and intima.

Along with skeletal muscle contraction, respiration also brings blood back to the heart. The diaphragm descends during inspiration, compressing abdominal veins. Intrathoracic pressure decreases during inspiration. Negative pressure draws air into the lungs and increases blood flow into the heart. The right atrium is within the thoracic cavity.

4.3.3 Capillaries

Capillaries are the major site of molecular exchange between the blood and extracellular fluid. Capillaries are the smallest blood vessels in the body and have diameters of 5–10 mm. They connect arterioles and venules and are also the blood vessels that most closely interact with tissues. Hence, they are the sites of nutrient transport to tissues. Capillaries are very thin and fragile, actually only one epithelial cell thick (Figure 4.6a). They are so thin that blood cells can only pass through them in single file (Figure 4.6b). Capillaries have no smooth muscle and so cannot dynamically change size to increase or decrease flow. Their diameter is less than that of a red blood cell, which is 7 micrometers in diameter. Capillaries, typically, are 5 micrometers at their inside diameter. The red blood cells must be distorted to pass through the capillaries.

Molecules cross the capillary wall through transcytosis (endocytosis and exocytosis), diffusion, and bulk flow (Figure 4.7). In transcytosis, molecules cross the epithelial cells through shuttling vesicles or vesicle-derived channels. There is also endocytosis, with phagocytosis as an example. This happens less frequently than transcytosis. Diffusion is the most important mechanism for exchange of water and dissolved substances. The rate of exchange can be up to 100 times higher than the rate of blood flow down a capillary. Molecules are able to diffuse across capillary walls by water-filled pores and through the cells. Pores are for slightly lipid soluble molecules, including Na^+, K^+, Cl^-, and glucose. More lipid soluble molecules, such as O_2, CO_2, and urea, diffuse through the endothelial plasma membranes. Water can use either mechanism.

The exchange of oxygen and carbon dioxide takes place through the thin capillary wall (Figure 4.8). The red blood cells inside of the capillary release their oxygen, which passes through the wall and into the surrounding tissue. The tissue releases its waste products, like carbon dioxide, which passes through the wall and into the red blood cells.

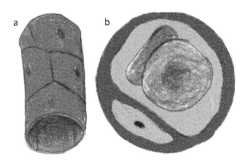

FIGURE 4.6 (a) A longitudinal section of a capillary and (b) a cross-section of a capillary with blood vessels, based on Figure by Berne, Levy, and Koeppen[1].

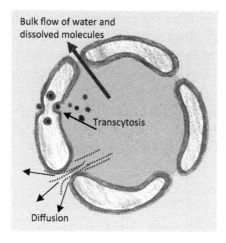

FIGURE 4.7 Movement across the capillary wall through transcytosis, diffusion, and bulk flow; based on Figure by Berne, Levy, and Koeppen[1].

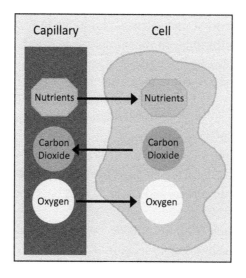

FIGURE 4.8 Movement from nutrients, carbon dioxide, and oxygen from capillary to cell.

The small diameter of the capillaries provides a large surface area for the exchange of gases and nutrients. In the lungs, carbon dioxide is exchanged for oxygen, whereas in the tissues, oxygen and carbon dioxide and nutrients (like glucose) and wastes are exchanged. In the kidneys, wastes are released to be eliminated from the body, and in the intestine, nutrients are picked up, and wastes released.

Capillaries are also involved in the release of excess heat. During exercise, your body and blood temperature rise, so to release excess heat, the blood delivers the heat to the capillaries which rapidly release it to the tissue (vasodilation). The result is that your skin takes on a flushed, red appearance.

Arteries and veins run parallel throughout the body, and the web-like network of capillaries, embedded in tissue, connects the two systems. The arteries pass their oxygen-rich blood to the capillaries, which allow the exchange of gases within the tissue. The capillaries then pass their waste-rich blood to the veins for transport back to the heart. The heart pumps blood out through the dorsal aorta. The main artery divides and branches out into many smaller arteries. Each region of your body has its own system of arteries supplying it with fresh, oxygen-rich blood.

The arteries deliver the oxygen-rich blood to the capillaries where the actual exchange of oxygen and carbon dioxide occurs. The capillaries then deliver the waste-rich blood to the veins for transport back to the lungs and heart.

4.4 BONE

The adult human body contains 206 bones. These bones provide structural support to the body and protect vital organs. These internal organs include the heart, lungs, and brain. Bones also serve as reserves for minerals such as calcium and house bone marrow-responsible for creating red blood cells (red marrow) and storing fat (yellow marrow).

Bones are composed mainly of a mineral phase and a fibrous protein phase. Calcium phosphate makes up a majority of the mineral present in bone. Hydroxyapatite, $Ca_{10}(PO_4)_6(OH)_2$, is the predominant calcium phosphate in mature bone. It has an elastic modulus of 114 GPa and is insoluble in water at physiological pH. This high-elastic modulus gives bone a high compressive strength. Mineralization (formation of a ceramic phase) of the collagen in bone results in stiffening of the tissue. This creates an increased ultimate tensile strength and compressive strength, lowers the strain at failure, and increases the elastic modulus. Therefore, as bone mineralizes, it can resist more force but is less ductile and more brittle (Figure 4.9).

The main type of protein in bone is type I collagen. Type I collagen is a fiber-forming protein that is the main load bearing element in numerous tissues such as blood vessels, skin, tendons, bone, ligament, cornea, and fascia. It gives bone toughness and some elasticity (a small amount).

Although they seem simple from the outside, bones have multiple levels of architectural complexity and are biologically complex[6] (Figure 4.10). To have enough strength to support your weight, but light enough to allow movement, bones (particularly long bones) have two types of architecture (Figure 4.10).

Cortical bone is the outer layer of bone. It is very dense, 5%–10% porous and makes up 10% of bone total surface area, but it is so dense that it makes up 80% of our skeletal bone

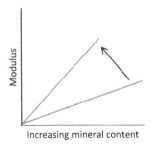

FIGURE 4.9 Increases in mechanical properties with increased mineralization.

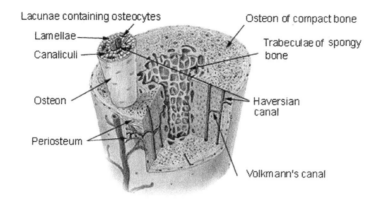

Lacunae containing osteocytes
Lamellae
Canaliculi
Osteon
Periosteum
Osteon of compact bone
Trabeculae of spongy bone
Haversian canal
Volkmann's canal

FIGURE 4.10 Cortical and trabecular bone. (From Wikimedia Foundation I. Osteon: Wikimedia Foundation; 2018. Available from: https://en.wikipedia.org/wiki/Osteon.)

mass. Cortical bone is primarily found on the outside of long bones, at the ends of joints, in vertebrae. Cortical bone is a complex material composed of a system of mineralized collagen fibers wrapped into spiral-like patterns forming a group of fused tubes, osteons, with canals, Haversian canals. Cortical bones have compressive strengths as high as 150 MPa and compressive moduli of up to 20 GPa.[7-9]

Beneath the cortical bone is the trabecular bone, also called *cancellous bone* or *spongy bone*. Trabecular bone is spongy is the inner porous structure of long bone, it makes up a majority of the bone volume but only 20% of skeletal bone mass. Its porosity makes it lightweight. The "spongy" look of trabecular bone is results from the arrangement of the spicules that organize it. Spicules are needle-like pieces of bone with large spaces between them. Trabecular bone is usually classified as "randomly organized," but after remodeling throughout the life span of an animal the spicules do develop a degree of organization. The spicules become more linearly aligned to support applied loads. Even with this arrangement, trabecular bone is still very porous and not very strong. Trabecular bones have compressive strengths up to 12 MPa and compressive moduli up to 5 GPa.[7-9] Trabecular bone makes up 20% of skeletal bone mass, and thus is very lightweight.

Although it is usually classified as randomly organized, trabecular bone can have some organization, which is created after remodeling, where cells begin to breakdown and rebuild the bone. The spicules are aligned in a way that best supports load. This means they become more linearly aligned. They still are very porous, so they lack strength.

Bone also contains several types of cells, and it houses other tissue types. Bones house blood vessels and nerve cells, primarily in the cortical bone. Bones also house osteocytes, which can differentiate into the two cell types responsible for bone remodeling, osteoclasts and osteoblasts. Osteoclasts break down old bone and osteoblasts build new bone. The inner bone cavities contain bone marrow, where red blood cells are produced. Red bone marrow is a soft tissue that produces blood cells, and yellow bone marrow is a store for fat. Bone consists of a mineral phase and a fibrous protein phase. The mineral phase is calcium phosphate, mainly in the form of hydroxyapatite. The mineral is rigid and gives the bone its compressive strength. The main type of protein in bone is type I collagen, which is flexible and gives bone toughness and some elasticity (a small amount).

4.4.1 Types of Bone

Bones are split into four categories. Long bones are found in your arms and legs, mostly made of compact bone. Short bones are in your wrists and ankles, mainly made of spongy bone. Flat bones make up your ribs and skull, made of a layer of spongy bone sandwiched between two thin layers of compact bone. The last type, irregular bones, includes the pelvis and other unusual shaped bones.

Bones are further classified as axial or appendicular, where axial bones are protective; for example, spinal vertebrae act to protect the spinal cord. Appendicular bones are the limbs. Note that the bones that make up the spinal column are unique.

There are three general forms of bone: woven, plexiform, and lamellar. Woven bone is a disorganized form of bone that is associated with youth (younger than age 5; Figure 4.11). Fetal bone is initially woven when it is first produced. Woven bone is also produced following damage as a result of trauma or disease. After a bone fracture, woven bone is produced to form a callus that keeps the broken bone together. It has few collagen fibers, randomly oriented, which gives woven bone low strength. Woven bone is unique in its ability to form spontaneously without a preexisting structure.

Lamellar bone is a type of secondary bone. It is produced from the remodeling of woven bone. It is produced more slowly than woven bone and is more organized than woven bone. It is produced in units called *lamellae*. The collagen fibers in lamellar bone have a parallel alignment; these aligned fibers form sheets called *lamellae*. These lamellae wrap around each other to form a tube called an *osteon* (Figures 4.10 and 4.12). The inside of the osteon is the Haversian canal. This alignment and the subsequent ordered mineral structure that it sponsors makes lamellar bone mechanically strong. Lamellar bone has much more collagen than woven bone.

Plexiform bone is formed more rapidly than primary or secondary lamellar bone tissue. It is primarily found in large, rapidly growing animals such as cows or sheep and is rarely

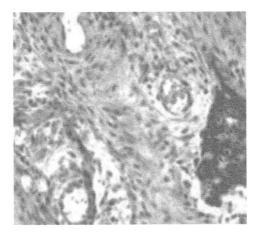

FIGURE 4.11 Scanning electron microscopy image of woven bone.

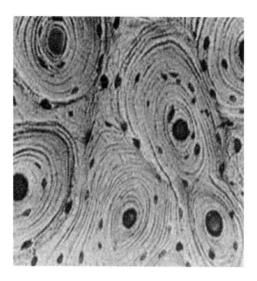

FIGURE 4.12 Scanning electron microscopy image of osteons of lamellar bone. (Courtesy of feppd.org.)

seen in humans. Plexiform bone obtained its name from the vascular plexuses contained within lamellar bone sandwiched by nonlamellar bone. Plexiform bone arises from mineral buds, which grow first perpendicular and then parallel to the outer bone surface. This produces the brick-like structure (Figure 4.13). Each "brick" in plexiform bone is about 125 microns across. Plexiform bone must be formed on existing bone or cartilage surfaces and cannot be formed de novo like woven bone. Because of its organization, plexiform bone offers much more surface area compared to primary or secondary bone upon which bone can be formed. This increases the amount of bone that can be formed in a given time frame and provides a way to more rapidly increase bone stiffness and strength in a short period of time. Although plexiform may have greater stiffness than primary or secondary cortical bone, it may lack the crack arresting properties which would make it more suitable for more active species like canines (dogs) and humans.

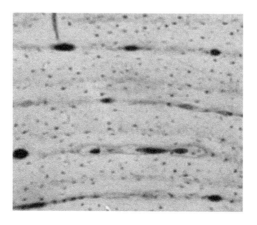

FIGURE 4.13 Scanning electron microscopy image of plexiform bone.

The periosteum is a sheet of fibrous connective tissue that covers bones. It has an inner layer of undifferentiated cells, rich with capillaries, and has the potential to form bone during growth and fracture healing. It is not present on all parts of the bone or on all bones. Periosteum is absent where tendons or ligaments join to the bone and also on cartilage-lined surfaces. It provides nutrients to the bone as well.

4.4.2 Human Bone Structure

The basic unit of bone is the Haversian system, which is comprised of a hollow, laminated rod of collagen and calcium phosphate; with a nutrient channel at the core (Haversian canal). Within the shaft of a long bone, many of these Haversian systems are bundled together in parallel, forming a kind of bone called *compact bone*, which is optimized to handle compressive and bending forces. Near the ends of the bones, where the stresses become more complex, the Haversian systems splay out and branch to form a meshwork of cancellous, or spongy, bone.

Lamallae consist of layers of mineralized collagen fibers that wrap around the Haversian canal (Figures 4.10 and 4.12). Layers range in thickness between 3 and 7 microns and are separated from each other by interlamellar layers. Osteons have diameters ranging from 200 to 300 microns. This central channel is called a *Haversian canal*, with a diameter of 50–90 microns. Within the Haversian canal is a blood vessel, typically 15 mm in diameter. Haversian canals contain nerve fibers and other bone cells called *bone-lining cells*. Bone-lining cells are actually osteoblasts, which have taken on a different shape following the period in which they have formed bone. If you cut a cross-section through a region of compact bone, you will see rings of Haversian systems, each with a hole, the canal, in the center. Cutting through the region of cancellous bone produces a more complex section because the systems have many different orientations.

There are three main structures present in lamellar cortical bone (the amounts of each can vary from bone to bone): circumferential lamellae, interstitial lamellae, and concentric lamellae that form the Haversian system. Circumferential lamellae are layers of lamellae that reach around the bone surface without interruption. Interstitial lamellae are angular pieces of circumferential or concentric osteons which fill the gaps of the Haversian system, and later become part of the cancellous bone system. Concentric lamellae are tubular structures that surround the central canal of osteons.

The Haversian system is made up of osteons, which is a group of concentric rings of bone (mineralized collagen) surrounding blood vessels. There are two types of osteonal tissue: primary and secondary. The primary osteonal cortical bone tissues are considered primary because they were there first. Primary osteons are formed in the absence of bone, formed from the mineralization of cartilage. There are few vascular channels and an even smaller number of lamellae. The second layer of cortical bone consists of the components of osteonal bone. Secondary osteons are formed through the remodeling of bone.

Osteocyte lacunae are ellipsoidal-shaped holes within bone that contain osteocytes and extracellular fluid. Their diameters are between 10 and 20 microns. Osteocyte canaliculi are the small tunnels that connect lacunae to one another. Osteocytes have processes that travel through the canaliculi to osteocytes in other lacunae. The processes in these tunnels may allow osteocytes within bone to communicate with one another to coordinate efforts to remodel bone.

Cement lines are boundaries in osteonal bone. They are less mineralized than the surrounding bone and are only 1–5 microns in thickness. They occur through bone remodeling and therefore, are only present in secondary bone. Cement lines are formed when bone resorption by osteoclasts ends and bone formation (by osteoblasts) begins. They are compliant and may absorb energy to stop cracks from growing in bone.

4.4.3 Bone Generation Cycle

In an adult, bone engages in a continuous cycle of breaking down and rebuilding. Bone-absorbing cells called *osteoclasts* break bone down and discard worn cells. After a few weeks, the osteoclasts disappear, and osteoblasts come to repair the bone. During the cycle, calcium is deposited and withdrawn from the blood.

4.5 LIGAMENT AND TENDON

Tendons and ligaments are multicomponent cable-like tissue that can cyclically transmit force without permanent dimensional changes (under normal physiological loads). These tissues translate muscle contraction into movement (tendons) and limit bone translation (ligaments). They are classified as *dense regular fibrous connective tissues.*

4.5.1 Ligament and Tendon Composition

Ligaments and tendons are dense, complex, and highly organized fibrous tissues composed of proteins called *collagens* (mainly types I with small amounts of III, and V) and *elastin.* Hyaluronic acid, proteoglycans (chondroitin sulfate and dermatan sulfate), water, and cells also comprise these tissues. Dermatan sulfate is found in orthogonal arrays around the collagen fibers that form fascicles. They bind specifically to the collagen d bands. The mechanical properties of tendon are a direct consequence of the constituent components and how these components are arranged. The collagen in these tissues is arranged in parallel bundles. These are multi-unit hierarchical structures that contain collagen molecules, fibrils, fibril bundles, fascicles, and tendon units that run parallel to the geometrical axis (Figure 4.14).[10]

Proteoglycans (PGs) in tendons and ligaments include decorin, a small leucine-rich PG. It binds specifically to the d band of positively stained type I collagen fibrils, which include

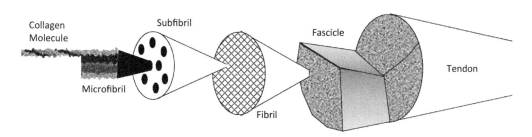

FIGURE 4.14 A diagram of tendon structure. (Based on a figure from Kastelic, J. et al., *Connect. Tissue Res.*, 6, 11–23, 1978.)

hyaluronan, a high molecular weight polysaccharide, biglycan, fibromodulin, lumican, epiphycan, and keratocan.

PGs are seen as filaments regularly attached to collagen fibrils. In relaxed mature tendons, most PG filaments are arranged orthogonally. They are located across the collagen fibrils at the gap zone, usually at the d and e positively staining bands. In immature tendons, PGs are observed either orthogonal or parallel to the D period. The amount of PGs associated with collagen fibrils in tendons decreases with increased fibril diameter and age.

Decorin regulates collagen fibril size and alignment. Animals lacking decorin have collagen fibrils with irregular diameters and decreased skin strength. Lumican controls collagen fibril size, so a model lacking lumican shows abnormally thick collagen fibrils and skin fragility. PGs such as decorin and other glycoproteins found in the ECM are required for normal collagen fibrillogenesis. Decorin also appears to facilitate fibrillar sliding during mechanical deformation.

4.5.2 Ligament and Tendon Structure and Behavior

Collagen fibers in ligaments and tendons are crimped. They display a change in direction that gives the fibers a wavy appearance, which is important for mechanical properties[11] (Figure 4.15). Ligaments (and tendons) are viscoelastic, which means that when under tension, they gradually lengthen. This is one reason why dislocated joints must be set as quickly as possible. If the ligaments lengthen too much, then the joint will be weakened, becoming prone to future dislocations.

4.5.3 Tendons

Tendons connect muscle to bone, transmitting forces generated by the muscle to the bone. Tendons are composed of collagen, elastin, proteoglycans, cells, and water. There are two tendons associated with every muscle: proximal tendons and distal tendons. The nutrient supply to tendons include blood vessels in the covering of the tendon, blood vessels in periosteal insertion, and blood vessels from surrounding tissues. It is interesting to note that tendon length is related to muscle size. Someone with 1-cm biceps tendon will have greater potential for muscle mass than someone longer tendons. Bodybuilders usually have short tendons.

Tendons are sometimes considered to be part of the muscle. The muscle belly is not the total muscle. The tendon is the "stroma," or supporting framework. The muscle belly is the "parenchyma." Together, the stroma and the parenchyma make up the muscle-tendon

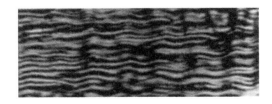

FIGURE 4.15 Crimp pattern of collagen in tendon. (Taken from McBridge, D.J., *Hind Limb Extensor Tendon Development in the Chick: A Light and Transmission Electron Microscopic Study*, Rutgers University, Newark, NJ, 1984.)

unit. The muscle-tendon unit is responsible for the movement of the skeletal system and the maintenance of joint stability. Joint stability is usually attributed to ligaments, which are actually backup to muscle-tendon units.

Tendons can be flat, cylindrical, and ribbon shaped. More powerful muscles have short and broad tendons (e.g., quadriceps). Muscles in charge of precise, subtle movements have long and thin tendons (finger flexors).

Myotendinous junction (MTJ) connects the tendon to muscle. The osteotendinous junction (OTJ) connects the tendon to bone. The origin is where muscle and tendon meet, and the enthesis is located where the tendon meets the bone. Here, the collagen fibers become mineralized and join the bone. In the tendon, collagen molecules combine to form fibrils. Collagen fibrils combine to form fibers, which are brought together to form fascicles surrounded by endotenon. The fascicles are combined to form a tendon, which is surrounded by epitendinium and paratenon. At the origin, collagen fibers extend from within the muscle and into the tendon. Collagen fibers are mineralized at the enthesis and integrated into the bone. Endotenon contains blood vessels, which are parallel to the collagen fibers and can branch occasionally.

The epitenon and peritenon contain nerve endings. Golgi tendon organs are present at the junction between tendon and muscle. Some tendons are surrounded by a sheath, namely fibrous sheaths (retinacula), found in hands and feet, and seen in tendons that move through grooves and notches. Paratenon is composed of loose collagenous fibrillar tissue, which allows movement of tendon against surrounding tissue. Epitenon is located beneath the paratenon and is composed of collagen fibrils 10-nm thick. Its fibers align with strain but do not completely align. Endotenon is composed of criss-crossed collagen fibers. PGs are endotenon and tendon fibers that hydrate the tendon. Endotenon allows fiber bundles to glide with respect to one another. They carry blood vessels, nerves, and lymphatics to the tendon.

The synovial sheath is located in tendons that do not have an epitendinium. It is a closed duct around tendons that glides on bone surfaces. The synovial sheath is seen in tendons of hand and feet and has two membranes: the inner (visceral) sheet and the outer (parietal) sheet. Synovial (peritendinous) fluid fills the space between parietal and visceral membranes and facilitates smooth gliding of the tendons. It also provides nutrition.

4.5.4 Ligament

Ligaments connect bone to bone. Capsular ligaments are part of the articular capsule that surrounds synovial joints, acting as mechanical reinforcements. Extracapsular ligaments join bones together and provide joint stability. Ligaments are similar to tendon in hierarchical structure. Collagen fibrils are slightly less in volume fraction and organization than in tendons. Ligaments also have a higher percentage of PG matrix than tendons do. They get nutrients through microvascularity from insertion sites.

Ligaments vary in size, shape, orientation, and location. They have bony attachments (insertions). Ligaments are surrounded by a more vascular layer (epiligament). The epiligament receives blood from an artery branch and is more cellular than the rest of the ligament and is also innervated (sensory and proprioceptive nerves). This layer merges into the periosteum of the bone around the attachment sites. Beneath the epiligament, the ligament is organized hierarchically into interconnected groups of parallel fibers known as *bundles*. In ligament, fibers appear to tighten or loosen depending on the bone positions and the forces that are applied. Fibers are not all aligned along the ligament long axis.

4.5.5 Ligament and Tendon Cells and Composition

Both tissues contain types of fibroblasts. Studies have indicated that ligament and tendon cells may communicate via cytoplasmic extensions. Gap junctions have also been detected in association with these cell connections. This raises the possibility of cell-to-cell communication and the potential to coordinate cellular and metabolic responses throughout the tissue.

Tendon fibers are parallel and twisting. Ligament fibers are arranged in parallel layers that are criss-crossed one on top of the other. This criss-cross layering neutralizes the inherent elasticity of the collagen. The only elasticity in ligaments comes from white elastic fibers between each layer of the ligament. These allow some movement between the layers, but do not make the ligament elastic. If ligaments were tight enough to stabilize joints, our movement would be inhibited. Ligaments lack great elasticity (<3% elastin). Their primary function is to keep a dislocated joint in place. They are used after the muscle-tendon unit has surpassed its limit. Ligaments only protect joints if the muscle-tendon units are breached. They act as backup to the muscle-tendon unit, so elasticity is not a desirable quality. During normal motion, ligaments remain lax.

Ligaments are composed of bundles of white fibrous tissue placed parallel, closely interlaced with one another. They have a white, shining silvery appearance. Ligaments are strong, tough, and not able to extend easily. They are not involved in stretching. The overall ligament is non-elastic. Elastin between the layers allows some change of motion, or direction. If they were all bound together, it would be an almost rigid structure. Tendons and ligaments have the same components but in different amounts (Table 4.1).[12]

There are four elastic ligaments: ligamentum flavum, broad ligament of the uterus, vocal chords, and suspensory ligaments in the lens. Ligamentum flavum is made from yellow elastic fibers. It runs through the entire spinal column, protects the spinal cord from the spinal column, and is a soft elastic curtain that gives all the movements of the spinal column. The broad ligament of the uterus holds the uterus in place. It has to stretch when the uterus expands. Vocal chords come in two sets: vocal ligaments and vocal muscles. Suspensory ligaments in the lens stretch when the eye muscles want to change the diameter of the lens.

TABLE 4.1   Tendon and Ligament Composition

Component	Tendon Composition	Ligament Composition
Collagen	70%–80%	75%–85%
Elastin	10%–15%	<3%
Proteoglycans	1%–3%	1%–2%

4.5.6 Ligament and Tendon Damage: Sprain Compared with Strain

A sprain is an injury to a ligament. Commonly injured ligaments are in the ankle, knee, and wrist. These are injured by being stretched too far from their normal position. Ligaments are not elastic (<3% elastin). Ligaments therefore prevent abnormal movements but do stretch and tear when moved too far. A strain is an injury to a muscle or tendon. Muscles are made to stretch, but if stretched too far, or if stretched while contracting, a strain may result. This means a stretching or tearing of the muscle or tendon.

A common sprain, the twisted ankle, results if you fall or step on an uneven surface and roll your foot to the inside. This stretches the ligaments on the outside of your ankle, notably the talofibular and calcaneofibular ligaments. Sprains are commonly graded according to the degree of the injury. Grade I and Grade II ankle sprains can usually be treated with treatments such as ice and physical therapy. Grade III ankle sprains can lead to permanent ankle instability, and surgery may be required.

4.6 SKIN

Your skin is the largest single organ in your body. It is 1.8 m² in surface area and 11 kg in weight; the average weight for a male in the United States is 87 kg. Skin is involved with functions critical to human viability. It provides a regenerative, self-healing barrier from physical, biological, and chemical attack/injury and external influence and is primarily responsible for maintaining internal homeostasis and water balance through thermoregulatory secretory activity. Skin provides a neurological vehicle to relay information about the external environment to the body through sensory reception. It also acts as a location for biochemical synthesis of essential vitamins and hormones.

Skin serves many purposes, from the protection of inner organs to temperature control and sensory control. To protect the rest of the body, the skin acts as a physical barrier between the internal and external environment. When it comes to fighting pathogens, Langerhans cells in the skin are part of the adaptive immune system. Sensation from the skin is attributed to nerve endings that react to heat, cold, touch, pressure, vibration, and injury. Heat regulation is made possible by skin's large blood supply, which is far greater than its requirements. This is necessary for control of energy (heat) loss by radiation, convection, and conduction. Dilated blood vessels increase perfusion and heat loss, whereas constricted vessels greatly reduce cutaneous blood flow and conserve heat.

The skin controls evaporation by providing a relatively dry and impermeable barrier to fluid loss. Loss of this function contributes to the massive fluid loss in burns. Skin plays an important role in aesthetics and communication. Others see our skin and can assess our mood, physical state, and attractiveness. Skin also acts as a storage center for lipids and water. Certain parts of the skin synthesize vitamins D and B using UV light. This is linked to pigmentation, with darker skin producing more vitamin B than D, and vice versa. The concentration of urea in skin is 1/130th that of urine (negligible amount).

Absorption is an important function of the skin. Oxygen, nitrogen, and carbon dioxide can diffuse into the epidermis in small amounts. Some animals use their skin for their sole respiration organ. The skin is an important site of transport in many other organisms. Medicine can be administered through the skin through ointments or by means of adhesive patches, such as the nicotine patch.

Skin is classified as a dense, irregular, fibrous connective tissue. Unlike tendon or ligament skin, it does not contain aligned collagen fibers. It is an alignable network of collagen fibers. The collagen in skin is not arranged in parallel bundles, unlike tendons and ligaments. To properly protect the organs underneath it, skin must be able to handle different loads from different directions.

4.6.1 Skin Components

Skin is a continuous mechanical matrix comprised mostly of extracellular tissue. It is a multilayered interwoven network of collagen and elastic fibers. It also contains specialized cells (squamous cells, melanocytes, etc.), specialized structures (hair follicles and sweat glands), and neural circuitry. The combination of these elements gives skin its structural and mechanical properties and makes it critical for normal function. The ability of skin to give shape to tissues is largely a consequence of the macromolecules within skin (elastin and collagen). The ability of skin to store, transmit, and dissipate mechanical energy associated with gravity or impact loads involves the collagen fibrils.

The skin's wet weight is comprised of approximately 60%–72% water, 30% collagen, 0.2% elastin, 0.03%–0.035% glycosaminoglycan, cellular components and noncollagenous, and proteins that also comprise a small fraction of the wet weight. Skin's dry weight is 70%–80% collagen, the most important structural component of skin. An interesting note, you produce less elastin and more collagen as you age. This is why skin begins to sag and wrinkle as we age.

Skin has two layers: the epidermis and dermis; there is also a layer below the skin (hypodermis or subcutis, or subcutaneous layer; Figure 4.16). Each layer has a distinct role in skin function. The epidermis is mainly a protective barrier, whereas the dermis is primary structural, physiological, neurological, and metabolic.

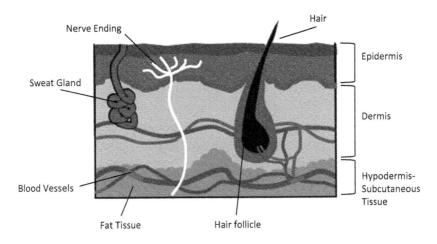

FIGURE 4.16 Drawing of the different layers of skin.

4.6.2 Epidermis

In skin, the epidermis is the superficial layer that provides waterproofing and a barrier to infection. It is composed of epithelial cells (live and dead) and keratin (inside of the cells). The epidermis is 10% of the total skin thickness. This varies from 0.1 mm at the eyelids to nearly 1 mm on the palms and soles. The outermost epidermis consists of stratified squamous epithelium. The epidermis contains no blood vessels. Cells in the deepest layers are nourished by diffusion from blood capillaries extending to the upper layers of the dermis.

In skin, the epidermis can be further subdivided into the following layers: stratum corneum, stratum lucidum, stratum granulosum, stratum spinosum, and stratum basale (Figure 4.17). The cells in the epidermis travel from the bottom to the surface, which means cells are formed at the basal layer. The cells move up the strata, changing shape and composition as they die because of isolation from their blood source. As they die, the cytoplasm is released, and the protein keratin is inserted. Cells eventually reach the corneum and slough off (desquamation). This process is called *keratinization* and takes place within about 30 days. This keratinized layer of skin is responsible for keeping water in the body and keeping other harmful chemicals and pathogens out. It makes skin a natural barrier to infection.

The main type of cells in the epidermis is the keratinocyte, with smaller numbers of melanocytes and Langerhans cells. Depending on their location, keratinocytes are called *basal* or *squamous cells*. Basal cells lie at the bottom of the epidermis. They are shaped like rounded columns. They divide and push older cells into higher layers. As the cells move into the higher layers, they flatten and eventually die.

Squamous cells are flat cells that look like fish scales. "Squamous" comes from the Latin squama meaning "the scale of a fish or serpent." These cells shed every 2 weeks. They are basal cells that have been flattened. Squamous cells make up most of the cells in the outer

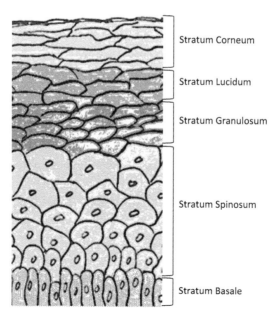

Stratum Corneum

Stratum Lucidum

Stratum Granulosum

Stratum Spinosum

Stratum Basale

FIGURE 4.17   Drawing of the different layers in the epithelium in skin.

layer of the skin (the epidermis), the passages of the respiratory, the lining of the digestive tract, and the linings of the hollow organs of the body.

Other cells include melanocytes, which produce melanin, a pigment that gives skin its color. They lie in deepest parts of the epidermis. Another type, Langerhans cells, serve as the frontline defense of the immune system in the skin. There are also Merkel's cells, whose function is not clearly known. Blood capillaries are found beneath the epidermis and are linked to an arteriole and a venule.

4.6.3 Dermis

The dermis is the underlying layer of skin. It contains collagen and elastic fibers, sweat glands, nerves, hair follicles, blood vessels, and fat (Figure 4.16). It is thickest at the palms, soles and back (3 mm), and thinnest at the eyelids (0.3 mm). The dermis is responsible for thermoregulation and supporting the vascular network. This supplies the avascular epidermis with nutrients. The dermis contains mostly fibroblasts, which are responsible for secreting collagen, elastin, and ground substance. These give the support and elasticity of the skin. Also present are immune cells that are involved in defense against foreign invaders passing through the epidermis.

The dermis consists of blood vessels, nerves, hair follicles, smooth muscle, glands, and lymphatic tissue. Specialized functions of the dermis are attributed to erector muscles attached between the hair papilla and epidermis, which can contract, resulting in the hair fiber pulled upright, and consequentially, the formation of goose bumps. Other special functions of the skin include the result of sebaceous glands, which produce sebum, a mixture of lipids and waxy substances for lubrication, water-proofing, and softening and antibactericidal actions, as well as sweat glands, which open up via a duct onto the skin by a pore.

The dermis contains loose connective tissue, primarily collagen, elastin, and reticular fiber, which is one or more types of very thin and delicately woven strands of collagen. Many of these types of collagen have been combined with carbohydrates.

The dermis can be subdivided into two layers: the superficial papillary layer and the reticular dermis. The papillary layer is outermost and extends into the epidermis to supply it with nutrients. It is composed of loosely arranged fibers, type I and III collagen fibers, and elastic fibers. These same proteins are found in the reticular layer. The maximum diameters of the collagen fibrils are 100 nm. Elastic fibers make up only 2% of the weight of this layer. It is interesting to note that papillary ridges make up the lines of the hands and feet, producing individually unique fingerprints and footprints.

The reticular layer is denser and continuous with the hypodermis. It contains the bulk of the specialized structures (sweat glands) and is composed of irregularly arranged fibers and resists stretching. The deep reticular layer represents about 75% of the skin by volume. It serves as the essential macromolecular support structure imparting skin with its overall strength and elasticity.

Collagen meshwork present in the dermis provides the bulk of the skin support structure's mechanical strength. Of the total collagen content in skin, 80% is type I collagen, whereas 15% is type III collagen. The remaining 5% are of other collagen types (IV, V, VI,

VII, XII, and XIV) contribute to the stability and performance of the ECM. The major function of collagen fibers and the structures they form are to prevent tissue failure by withstanding deformation and dissipating energy. Collagen fibers form a non-woven network of wavy collagen fibers. These fibers allow the skin to maintain its shape when loads are removed. The fibers align in the direction of the applied stress.

4.6.4 Hypodermis

The hypodermis is actually a subcutaneous adipose tissue layer and is also called the *basement membrane*. It attaches skin to the underlying bone and muscle and supplies the dermis with blood vessels and nerves (Figure 4.16). The hypodermis insulates the body by padding it (shock absorber) and acting as a caloric reserve. It consists of loose connective tissue, elastin, and fat. The main cell types are fibroblasts, macrophages, and adipocytes. The hypodermis contains 50% of body fat. Microorganisms like *Staphylococcus epidermidis* colonize the skin surface. These microorganisms serve as a form of protection against disease. The disinfected skin surface gets recolonized from bacteria residing in the deeper areas of the hair follicle.

4.7 CARTILAGE

Cartilage is a type of dense connective tissue that is composed of collagen fibers or elastic fibers and contains cells called *chondrocytes*. The fibers and cells are embedded in a firm gel-like ground substance called the *matrix* that is mainly made up of PGs. It is enclosed in a dense connective tissue called the *perichondrium*. The perichondrium is a dense membrane composed of fibrous connective tissue that closely wraps all cartilage, except the cartilage in joints, which is covered by a synovial membrane. Cartilage is an avascular tissue so cellular nutrients are diffused through the matrix. This makes sense because structurally cartilage usually subjected to lots of stress. If the tissue was rich with blood vessels they would become damaged, leading to tearing and clotting.

Cartilage serves several functions. It provides a framework for bone deposition to begin. Cartilage supplies a smooth surface for the movement of articulating bones. It also provides shock absorption between neighboring bones. Cartilage is found in joints, the rib cage, ear, nose, bronchial tubes, and between intervertebral discs.

Cartilage is composed of collagen fibers (primarily type II, with smaller amounts of types V, VI, IX, X, and XI), elastic fibers (in elastic cartilage), PGs (and glycosaminoglycans), water, cells (chondrocytes), and ions (the predominant ions within the interstitial fluid are sodium, chloride, potassium, and calcium).[13]

Chondrocytes are the only cells found in cartilage; their precursors are chondroblasts. Chondrocytes are responsible for the secretion and maintenance of the matrix. They lie within spaces called *lacunae* and exist singly or in groups called *cell nests* (Figure 4.18).[14]

In general, the matrix is composed of PGs. PGs are large molecules with a protein backbone and glycosaminoglycan (GAG) side chains. The most common types of GAGs in cartilage are chondroitin sulfate and keratan sulfate. The matrix immediately surrounding the chondrocytes is referred to as the *territorial matrix*, or *capsule*. Water is the most abundant component of articular cartilage. It is believed that in normal cartilage approximately 30%

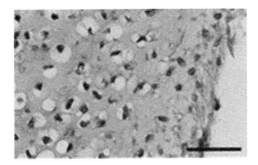

FIGURE 4.18   Chondrocytes in lacunae. (From Tsuchida, A.I. et al., *Arthritis Res. Ther.*, 16, 441, 2014.)

of the water lies within the intrafibrillar space of collagen. The diameter of collagen fibers is modulated by the swelling pressure generated by the "fixed charge density" (FCD) of the surrounding PGs. The amount of water within the intrafibrillar compartment is controlled by the FCD. Water gets into the fibers and increases the density through swelling. The degree of collagen fiber swelling is also controlled by crosslinks; more crosslinks lead to less swelling.

In the native tissue, it appears that most of this intrafibrillar water is not available for transport under mechanical loading and is excluded from the PGs and bound to the collagen. This exclusion effectively raises the density of the fixed charges within the tissue. This, in turn, raises the interstitial osmotic pressure and charge-charge repulsion, which increases the efficiency of cartilage as a shock absorber.

In contrast, there is a significant increase of water content in degenerating articular cartilages. In cartilage from osteoarthritic joints, disruption of the collagen network can cause the water content of the tissue to increase by more than 10%. This increase is not necessarily proteoglycan related. This is a result of the disruption of the collagenous matrix. The damaged collagen network is not able to restrain the swelling pressure produced by the GAG; more water comes in and volume increases.

The amount of water present in cartilage depends largely on the concentration of the PGs, FCD, resultant swelling pressure exerted by the negative charge groups on the PGs and ions dissolved in the interstitial fluid, and the organization of the collagen network. Intact matrices control tissue volume by limiting the degree to which the tissue can swell; this limits water content. The strength and stiffness of this network surrounding the PG molecules allows it to resist the swelling pressure. Most of the fluid and ions within the tissue are freely exchangeable by diffusion with the bathing solution surrounding the tissue. The interstitial fluid may also be extruded from the tissue by applying a pressure gradient across the tissue or by simply compressing the tissue.

4.7.1 Types of Cartilage

There are three different types of cartilage, each with special characteristics adapted to local needs hyaline, elastic, and fibrocartilage. Hyaline cartilage is the most abundant type of cartilage. It lines the edges of bones in joints. The word *hyaline* is derived from the Greek word *hyalos*, meaning "glass"; this refers to the translucent matrix (bluish white color). In hyaline cartilage, type II collagen makes up 40% of its dry weight, and it is arranged in cross-striated fibers, ranging from 15 to 45 nm in diameter. These fibers do not assemble into large bundles.

4.7.1.1 Hyaline Cartilage

Hyaline cartilage is primarily composed of type II collagen; it is extremely strong, very flexible, and elastic. Its chondrocytes are far apart from one another in fluid-filled lacunae.

Hyaline cartilage exists in:

- The trachea
- The larynx
- The tip of the nose
- The connection between the ribs
- The breastbone
- The ends of bone where they form joints (articular cartilage)
- Inside bones

Hyaline cartilage also serves as a center of ossification or bone growth and forms most of the embryonic skeleton. This later develops into primary osteonal bone. This is why babies have soft skeletons, which is necessary for birth. This allows the body of the child to be compressed while it travels through the birth canal without harming it or the mother.

Hyaline cartilage has several functions. Where it is found at the ends of articulating bones, it reduces friction at joints, facilitating bone movement. Hyaline cartilage joins bones firmly together in such a way that a certain amount of movement is still possible between them. Hyaline cartilage forms the c-shaped cartilaginous rings in the trachea and bronchi to assist in keeping those tubes open. It is responsible for the longitudinal growth of bone in the neck regions of the long bones.

Articular cartilage is a specialized hyaline cartilage. Its composition differs with age, site in the joint, and depth from the surface (Figure 4.19).[15] Normal articular cartilage contains 60%–70% collagen and 5%–15% PGs on a dry-weight basis. It is divided into four zones: the superficial zone, intermediate, deep zone, and calcified zone (Figure 4.20).[16]

The composition and structure of each zone is different. They have different mechanical properties. The collagen content is highest at the superficial layer and comprises about 10% of the cartilage thickness. The middle zone comprises about 60% of the cartilage thickness, and the deep zone comprises about 30% of the thickness. All cartilage tissues have distinctive lacunae.

In the superficial layer, there are no perichondrium on articulating bones. Groups of fine type II collagen fibrils anchor the PG matrix to bone. The collagen content is highest in the superficial layer. In the intermediate and superficial zones, the fibril bundles are composed of a fine meshwork of collagen fibrils that run at angles or parallel with respect to the surface. It comprises about 10% of the cartilage thickness.

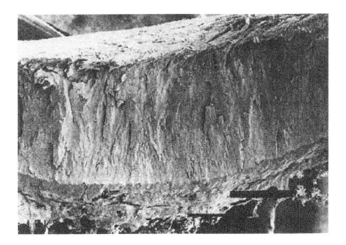

FIGURE 4.19 Scanning electron micrograph of articular cartilage. (From Wilson, W. et al., *Osteoarthritis Cartilage*, 14, 1196–1202, 2006.)

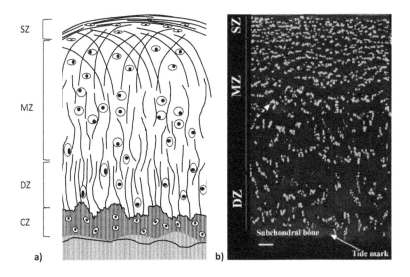

FIGURE 4.20 (a) Diagram of cells within articular cartilage and (b) a live-dead stain of chondrocytes within articular cartilage. (From Karim, A. et al., *J. Anat.*, 232, 686–698, 2018.) The cells in (b) follow the structure seen in (a). CZ calcification zone; DZ, deep zone; MZ, medial zone; SZ, superficial zone.

The middle zone comprises about 60% of the cartilage thickness. In the calcified and deep zones, the fibrils are arranged in vertical bundles with adjacent bundles closely connected with bridging fibrils. The deep zone comprises about 30% of the thickness of cartilage.

The deep and calcified zones are separated by the tidemark (a narrow band of mineral aggregates associated with matrix vesicles). The calcified zone forms the interface between cartilage and underlying subchondral bone. The subchondral bone serves to transmit loads from the cartilage into the underlying cancellous bone. The fluid content is about 85% at the surface and remains constant for about 25% of the depth. It falls to below 75% for the remaining portion of the cartilage.

4.7.1.2 Elastic Cartilage

Elastic cartilage is also called *yellow cartilage*. It is found in the pinna of the ear, where it maintains shape and flexibility, and in the walls of the auditory canals, eustachian canals, and larynx where it keeps these tubes open. Elastic cartilage contains type II collagen and elastic fibers. Elastic cartilage is similar to hyaline cartilage but contains a network of elastic bundles (elastin) scattered throughout the matrix that run through the matrix in all directions (Figure 4.21).[17]

4.7.1.3 Fibrocartilage

Fibrocartilage, also called *white cartilage*, is a tough tissue. It does not have the same underlying structure that is present in hyaline cartilage. Unlike the other cartilages, fibrocartilage contains type I collagen; overall it contains more collagen than hyaline cartilage and is composed of fibrous connective tissue arranged in parallel bundles (for increased tensile properties); chondrocytes lie between the bundles (Figure 4.22).[18] The orientation of the bundles depends upon the stresses acting on the cartilage. In some cases, fibrocartilage is produced when there is significant damage to cartilage and the underlying bone. The collagen bundles are aligned in the direction of the stress applied to it. In other cases, it is found in areas requiring tough support or great tensile strength such as the intervertebral discs, space between the pubic bones in front of the pelvic girdle, connections between ligaments and bone and tendons and bone, and around the edges of the articular cavities such as the glenoid cavity in the shoulder joint. In the connections between tendon and ligament and bone the fibrocartilage acts as a transition between the soft tissue (tendon/ligament) and hard tissue (bone), helping to keep joints together. Fibrocartilage

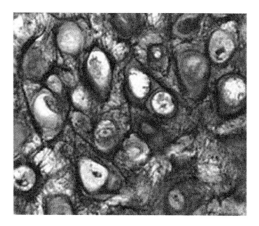

FIGURE 4.21 Picture of chondrocytes in elastic cartilage. Chondrocytes in lacunae lie among dark elastic fibers. (Taken from King, D., Elastic cartilage, http://www.siumed.edu/~dking2/ssb/NM011b.htm, 2009.)

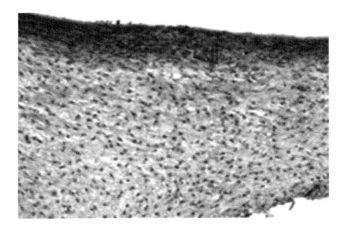

FIGURE 4.22 Fibrocartilage from a bone grafting procedure after Safranin-O and Fast-Green staining. (From Auffarth, A., *Am. J. Sports Med.*, 46, 1039–1045, 2018.)

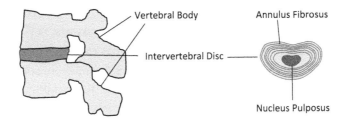

FIGURE 4.23 Drawing of the intervertebral disc and vertebral bodies.

also deepens ball and socket joints such as hips and shoulders. For both of these reasons, fibrocartilage helps to prevent joint dislocation.

The intervertebral disc (IVD) is located in the spine between vertebral bodies (Figure 4.23); there are 24 discs in the human spine. In the IVD, the fibrocartilage forms the annulus fibrosus that is arranged in layers (lamellae) and acts as a shock absorber preventing the vertebrae from contacting each other during impact and resists the stress from inside of the disc. The structure also protects the spinal cord from injury. The tissue absorbs shocks that would damage vertebrae during locomotion. The annulus fibrosus wraps around the nucleus pulposus, preventing it from coming out of the disc.

It also acts as a hinge to allow movement of the spine. The IVD has thick annulus fibrosus on the outside, a gel-like nucleus pulposus on the inside, and two vertebral end plates. The cartilaginous material in the annulus fibrosus is arranged in concentric lamellae, approximately 11–20 layers across. It is thicker in the anterior and lateral sections as well as toward the center, while thinner posteriorly (finer and more tightly packed). This makes sense mechanically; compression by vertebrae increases internal pressure, and the rings of collagen contain pressure by means of preventing expansion or bursting.

Our body weight is carried by discs. Vertebral bodies press on these discs, and with each step, the nucleus pulposus squishes down and out against the annulus fibrosus. The pressure is then transferred to the annulus fibrosus and forces it out.

Collagen fibers in each lamellae are parallel to one another and oriented at an angle off of the vertical axis. The end plate consists of both hyaline and fibrocartilage. Hyaline is located around the vertebral body and is more evident in neonatal and young discs. Fibrocartilage is located around the nucleus pulposus. Note that discs are almost all fibrocartilage in older discs.

The meniscus is also considered to be fibrocartilage. Menisci are semilunar cartilaginous structures that deepen and cushion the femoro-tibial articulation. It turns the tibial surface into a shallow socket to increase the stability of the knee joint. The meniscus spreads out the weight being transferred from the femur above to the tibia below; this protects the articular cartilage from excessive forces occurring in any one area on the joint surface. Without the meniscus, the round femur would slide on top of the flat tibial surface and the concentration of force onto a small area on the articular cartilage would damage the surface, leading to osteoarthritis. The meniscus is composed of 75% water and 25% collagen type I fibers, PGs, and chondrocytes. The architecture of the collagen fiber bundles is approximately parallel and is mainly circular in the thick peripheral portion of the meniscus. At the inner part of the meniscus, their orientation is mainly radial. The collagen fibers run parallel to the surface at the superficial layers and continue this trend but run radial too in the deeper layers. There are blood vessels in the peripheral zone. The larger part of the meniscus is avascular.

When the hyaline cartilage is damaged, it is often replaced with fibrocartilage. This typically happens at the knee, specifically at the end of the femur, but fibrocartilage does not withstand weightbearing forces as well as hyaline cartilage. The amount of fibrocartilage in the body increases with age. Hyaline cartilage "transforms" into fibrocartilage, meaning that it is more likely replaced with fibrocartilage after damage from years of stress. This is what happens in microfracture surgery. The subchondral bone underneath is cracked, releasing blood and cells into the damaged area, and these cells produce fibrocartilage to heal the newly formed defect. This is only a temporary fix and is synonymous to scar tissue. Different fiber arrangements between the tissues means different mechanical properties. Fibrocartilage is better under tension, whereas hyaline cartilage is better under compression.

4.7.2 Osteoarthritis

Osteoarthritis (OA) is the most prevalent musculoskeletal disease in humans, affecting nearly 21 million Americans. It causes pain, loss of joint motility and function, and severely reduces the standard of living of the patient. OA is a degenerative joint disease characterized by the breakdown of joint cartilage and predominately strikes adults older than age 45. Factors such as genetics, repetitive movement, trauma, and weight contribute to abnormal chondrocyte function and increased cartilage breakdown. OA can occur as a primary or secondary disorder, both of which are characterized by degeneration and loss of articular cartilage. Primary OA (idiopathic) is considered to be the result of insidious age-related "wear and tear" processes, whereas secondary OA develops following acute trauma. In both processes, disease is associated with excessive biomechanical stress.

Early events in the onset of OA include loss of PG from the cartilage ECM, disruption of the collagen network (leads to increased cartilage hydration), and decreased chondrocyte density. Decreased chondrocyte density and cell death have also been suggested as causal factors in the initiation of cartilage degradation. In normal healthy cartilage, chondrocytes are well protected from death by the integrity of their surrounding matrix. This protection is compromised when the matrix is damaged. Chondrocyte death is mainly thought to be initiated by matrix degradation. Cell death potentially causes further matrix degeneration through the release of degradative enzymes and reduction of matrix synthesis (no maintenance). Chondrocytes can respond to mechanical and/or chemical signals to increase production of matrix metalloproteinases (MMP), proinflammatory cytokines, and reactive oxygen species (ROS) and reactive nitrated oxygen species (RNS; nitric oxide [NO]). Abnormal cartilage loading may trigger the synthesis of all of these mediators, causing further damage to the matrix.

4.8 NERVOUS TISSUE

Nervous tissue regulates and coordinates many bodily activities. It detects and responds to changes in the internal and external environments and allows for states of consciousness, learning, memory, and emotions. Nervous tissue is designed to convert stimuli into electrical signals, transfer these signals to the processing center, process the signals, and stimulate tissues and organs based on those signals. The central nervous system, peripheral nervous system, brain, and spinal cord are nervous tissues. Like the other tissues that we have discussed, the function of nervous tissues in the neural system are predicated on the molecules that they are composed of; the main difference lies in function. These tissues contain two types of cells, neurons and neuroglia. Neurons are cells that can conduct impulses. Neurons have cell bodies, which houses the nucleus and other organelles; extensions from the cell body include the dendrites and the axon (Figure 4.24). Dendrites allow the neuron to send and receive signals through neuron-to-neuron connections called *synapses*. The axon also extends from the cell body and is used to make connections with other neurons using the axon terminals. The axon terminals come into close proximity to dendrites and exchange neurotransmitters, which pass the signal from the axon terminal

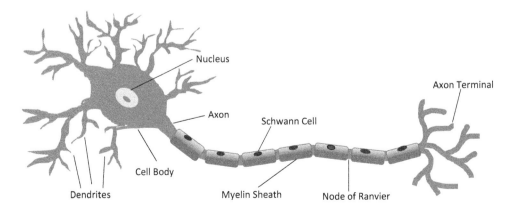

FIGURE 4.24 Structure of a neuron.

to the dendrites. From here, the signal travels down the axon of the neuron that received the signal through its dendrites and to the axon terminals. Neurons have different-sized axons depending on their job. Local circuit neurons or interneurons in the brain have shorter axons; projection neurons can have lengths of up to a meter depending on the target, like those that run from the spine to the foot.[19] The signal passes from the dendrite, down the axon, to the axon terminals using action potential. Action potentials send electrical impulses down the length of an axon through the movement of ions into the cell through ion gates. An action potential is a fast increase and decrease in voltage across the membrane of a cell.

4.8.1 Neuroglia

Neuroglia support and nourish neurons, there are far more neuroglia than neurons. Among the neuroglia are Schwann cells. These neuroglia cells increase the speed of the impulse down the length of the axon by myelinating it, producing a medullary sheath (Figure 4.24). This sheath is not continuous because it is interrupted by spaces called the *nodes of Ranvier* (Figure 4.24). The myelin sheaths increase electrical resistance across the cell membrane by a factor of 5,000 and decreases capacitance by a factor of 50. Myelin is a mixture of lipids (70%–80%) and proteins (20%–80%) that form around the nerve fibers, giving them a white appearance. Oligodendrocytes also myelinate axons (Figure 4.25). Oligodendrocytes interact with neurons in the central nervous system (CNS), whereas Schwann cells myelinate neurons in the peripheral nervous system (PNS).

Astrocytes are star-shaped neuroglia that are present in the spinal cord and brain (CNS). They supply nutrients to neurons, physically support neurons, repair damaged nervous tissue, bind neurons to capillaries, and maintain the blood-brain barrier (Figure 4.26). Astrocytes facilitate some communication between neurons by wrapping around neural synapses and through the release of neurotransmitters such as glutamate. Ependymal cells are ciliated neuroglia that are found within the walls of ventricles (cavities) in the brain and in the spinal cord (Figure 4.27). In the ventricles, the ependymal cells secrete cerebrospinal fluid (CSF), which surrounds the brain protecting it from physical injury and removing toxins from around the brain, depositing them into the bloodstream.

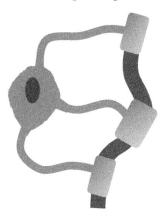

FIGURE 4.25   Oligodendrocyte linked to a neuron.

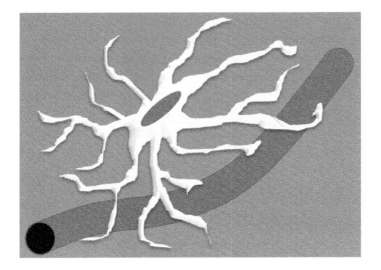

FIGURE 4.26   An astrocyte bound to a capillary.

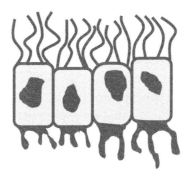

FIGURE 4.27   Ependymal cells that line ventricle walls in the brain and spinal cord central canal.

Satellite cells are similar to astrocytes except that they lie in the PNS, whereas astrocytes are in the CNS (Figure 4.28). Satellite cells surround, support, and protect neurons. Radial glia can spawn new neurons and help to move neurons to different places in the brain (Figure 4.29).

4.8.2 Spinal Cord

The spinal cord is a long cord composed of neurons that begins at the base of the brain, the medulla oblongata, and ends near the bottom of the spine. These nerves take signals to and from the brain. The spinal cord is surrounded by three layers of tissue called the *meninges*. The layers are called the *pia matter*, the *arachnoid matter*, and the *dura matter*. The spinal cord and surrounding meninges sit within the spinal canal in the center of the spine.

If you take a cross-section of the spinal cord you see a gray "butterfly-shaped" area surrounded by a whitish material (Figure 4.30). The gray area is gray matter that is made up of the cell bodies of the neurons that make up the spinal cord. The whitish area is the white matter that is made up of bundles of axons that travel down the cord and out to muscles from the brain (descending tracts) or up the cord from other parts of the body delivering

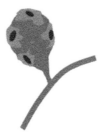

FIGURE 4.28   Satellite cell found in peripheral nervous system.

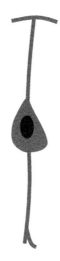

FIGURE 4.29   Drawing of a radial cell.

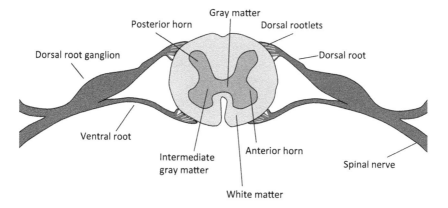

FIGURE 4.30   A schematic of the spinal cord displaying the spinal nerve, white matter, and gray matter.

sensory information to the brain (ascending tracts). These axons are myelinated, which is why they have a white appearance. The bundles are called *funiculi*.

In the gray matter, the anterior horns contain the motor neurons that send signals from the brain or spinal cord to stimulate skeletal muscle. The posterior horns contain the sensory neurons that transmit sensory information from other parts of the body to the brain and interneurons that connect with other neurons in the spinal cord. Between the anterior and posterior horns lies the intermediate gray matter. This area contains a mixture of neurons with diiferent tasks. Because its boundaries are not well developed, the intermediate gray matter has the cell bodies of some neurons (and interneurons) that stimulate skeletal muscle (as seen in the anterior horn) and some the cell bodies of some neurons (and interneurons) that transmit sensory information to the brain (from the posterior horn). The intermediate gray matter also contains cell bodies of neurons that regulate organs that are under involuntary control, heart, stomach, intestines, etc.

The motor neurons exit the spinal cord in ventral rootlets that come together to form a ventral root. The sensory neurons are organized in a similar manner, from the spinal cord they split into dorsal rootlets and come together to form dorsal roots. A little further down the cell bodies of the sensory neurons come together to form the dorsal root ganglion. Further down the dorsal root and ventral root combine to form the spinal nerve.

4.8.3 The Brain

The brain is a collection of neurons and neuroglia. Like the spinal cord it is protected by protective layers of tissue called the *meninges*. The outermost layer of the meninges is the dura matter; the dura matter is also split into two layers, the periosteum (which comes into contact with the skull) and the dura. The next layer is the arachnoid, which lies between the dura and the pia matter. The arachnoid is elastic in nature and contains blood vessels. The layer of the meninges closest to the brain is the pia matter. The brain is split into several different sections that coordinate the functions of different parts of the body and control aspects of informational comprehension, language, and personality (Figure 4.31).

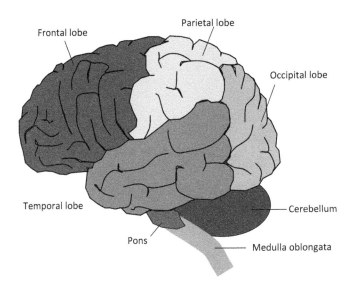

FIGURE 4.31 The different sections of the brain, including the four lobes.

4.8.3.1 Brainstem

The brainstem is the lower extension of the brain that is connected to the spinal cord. It is made up of the midbrain, pons, and medulla oblongata. It transfers signals back and forth between various parts of the body and the cerebral cortex. Eye movement and facial motor control are coordinated in the midbrain, whereas bladder control, eye movement, respiration, hearing, and balance are coordinated by the pons.[3,20] The medulla oblongata controls some reflexes, swallowing, respiration, and the cardio-vascular system (blood pressure and heart beats).[3,20] The thalamus aids in alertness and sleep patterns by coordinating motor and sensory signals traveling to the cerebral cortex.

4.8.3.2 Cerebellum

The cerebellum is on the bottom at the back of the brain. It is separated from the cerebrum by the tentorium (fold of dura). The cerebellum coordinates fine mtor movements and balance by controlling muscle tone.

4.8.3.3 Cranial Nerves

There are 12 pairs of nerves that originate directly from the brain itself and are responsible for swallowing and taste (vagus), movement of the tongue (hypoglossal), swallowing and taste (glossopharyngeal), smell (olfactory), eyelid movement, facial movement (facial), expression; taste sensation eye movement (abducens), sight (optic), eye and eyelid movement (oculomotor), eye movement (trochlear), neck and shoulder control (accesory), hearing and balance (vestibular), and facial senses (trigeminal).

4.8.3.4 Cerebrum

The cerebrum is split into a right and left hemisphere. The hemispheres are joined by a dense bundle of nerve fibers called the *corpus callosum*. The corpus callosum allows signals to be sent from one hemisphere to the other. The cerebral cortex lies at the top layer of the cerebrum. This area coordinates cognition, learning, memory, sensory perception, volunteer movement, and motor planning.[3,20] It has a wrinkled gray appearance (called *gray matter*). Beneath the cerebral cortex are connecting fibers between neurons called the *white matter*.[20] The wrinkles of the cerebral cortex consist of sulci (small grooves), fissures (larger grooves), and gyri (bulges between grooves).[20]

The cerebral hemispheres can be split into large regions called *lobes* by tracing along distinct fissures. The cerebrum is divided into pairs of frontal, temporal, parietal, and occipital lobes (one in each hemisphere).

4.8.3.5 Lobes of the Brain

The areas in the frontal lobes are responsible for speech, voluntary muscle movement, and behavior. Specifically, the prefrontal cortex is necessary for memory, intelligence, concentration, temper, and personality. Broca's area is in the left hemisphere frontal lobe, it controls facial muscles, tongue, and jaw and throat movement for language The premotor cortex in the frontal lobe coordinates head and eye movement.[3,20]

The occipital lobes take in and process visual information including processing shapes and colors. The lobe on the right hemisphere receives signals from the left side and the lobe on the left hemisphere receives signals from the right side.[20]

The parietal lobes interpret simultaneously signals received from other areas of the brain and processes information including signals for vision, temperature, taste, touch, hearing, motor, sensory, and memory.[20]

The temporal lobes are further divided into ventral (bottom) and lateral (side) sections. The right side aids in visual memory and recognition, the left side is involved in verbal memory for recalling understanding language, Wernicke's area is in the left temporal lobe; it allows people to make meaningful sounds (words). The back of the lobe is used to interpret emotions.[3,20]

4.8.3.6 Thalamus and Pituitary Gland

The thalmus is split into the hypothalamus, the epythalamus, the ventral thalamus, and the dorsal thalamus; the basal ganglia is around the thalamus. Information goes through the thalamus before going to the cortex. The thalamus controls motor relay and sensory relay to the cerebral cortex; it is involved in alertness and feeling pain. The hypothalamus controls the pituitary gland based on signals that it receives from the autonomic nervous system. The pituitary gland is joined to the bottom of the brain and controls hormone secretion.

4.8.4 Response to Injury

If axons are severed, neurons can regrow them. The axon segment that is separated from the cell body degenerates and sprouting begins at the portion connected to the cell body (proximal stump) and the new axon develops in the same direction as the original axon (if the route is clear). If the Schwann cells on the severed axon survive, they can guide the regeneration of the new axon through them to the original terminal site. The growth cone of the developing axon finds the Schwann cells allowing them to innervate the original target.[3,19] Return of function following a peripheral nerve injury is slow because axon regrowth occurs at approximately 1 mm per day.[19]

Although it is protected by layers of both hard and soft tissue, the spinal cord can be damaged. In most cases, the injury to the spinal cord is a bruise or crush, which leaves axons and connections physically intact as opposed to an injury that severs the cord. These types of injuries can lead to apoptosis of the oligodendrocytes. As the oligodendrocytes myelinate the axons, the loss of these cells results in the removal of myelin from the axons, which severely hampers the transmission of signals along the spinal cord. Sprouting occurs in the CNS, but the developing axons cannot find their original paths because the living oligodendrocytes that myelinate the cells are responsible for many neurons, not just one as seen in Schwann cells. Severed axons within the spinal cord may grow small new extensions but significant regeneration across the injury site is rarely seen.

Researchers are trying a variety of ways to provide an environment that will support axonal regeneration in the central nervous system. Most research revolves around the use of tubes to support regrowth of the severed axons, redirecting the axons to regions of the spinal cord that lack growth-inhibiting factors. This prevents apoptosis of the oligodendrocytes, so myelin can be maintained and signals transmitted effectively. Other groups are supplying neurotrophic factors that support recovery of the damaged tissue. In the brain, researchers are looking to stem cells to differentiate into new neurons to repopulate damaged areas in the brain.

4.9 MUSCLE

There are three types of muscle found in vertebrates: skeletal, cardiac, and smooth.[2,21] Cardiac muscle is found in the walls of the heart. Smooth muscle is present in the walls of all the hollow organs, including blood vessels (not the heart). Smooth muscle contraction reduces the size of the structures. Smooth muscle enables control of blood flow, moves food through gastrointestinal tract, forces urine from the bladder, contracts uterus during child birth, and regulates air flow through the lungs. The contraction of smooth muscle is generally not under voluntary control. Skeletal muscle is attached to the skeleton; it is also called *striated muscle*. Skeletal muscle is responsible for limb movement its contraction is under voluntary control.

4.9.1 Skeletal Muscle

A single skeletal muscle, such as the triceps muscle, is attached at the origin to a large area of bone via a tendon (Figure 4.32). At its other end, the insertion, it tapers into a tendon, which is attached to another bone. Some skeletal muscles are organized into two groups, extensors and flexors (Figure 4.32). These muscles work together they make an antagonistic pair of muscles. This pairing is necessary for skeletal movement because skeletal muscle

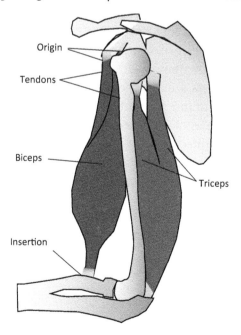

FIGURE 4.32 Drawing of two antagonistic muscles, biceps and triceps including tendons, the origin, and the insertion points.

exerts force only when it contracts. Therefore, you need antagonistic groups that will pull the limb in opposite directions to gain back and forth motion. An example of an antagonistic pair is the grouping of the triceps and biceps muscles. When the triceps contracts, the insertion is pulled toward the origin and the arm is straightened or extended at the elbow; the triceps is an extensor. The biceps muscle is the flexor of the lower arm; it flexes or bends the joint.

Skeletal muscle is made up of thousands of cylindrical muscle fibers (myofibers) often running all the way from origin to insertion. They are arranged in parallel. The fibers are bound together by connective tissue through which run blood vessels and nerves. A myofiber is a multinucleated single muscle cell (Figure 4.33).[22] Myofibers are formed when myoblasts (the single nuclei muscle cells) are fused together. The cell is densely packed with contractile proteins, energy stores, and signaling mechanisms. The myofiber is the smallest complete contractile system. Each muscle fiber contains a sarcolemma (plasma membrane), sarcoplasmic reticulum (endoplasmic reticulum), sarcosomes (mitochondria), and sarcoplasm (cytoplasm). The nuclei and mitochondria are located just beneath the plasma membrane.

The myofibers are embedded in a matrix of collagen. At either end of the muscle belly, the matrix becomes the tendon that connects the muscle to bone (Figure 4.32). The tissue gradually increases in collagen content and decreases in muscle content until it becomes the tendon (Figure 4.32). The change happens gradually, so the tendon and muscle are considered to be one unit. It is believed that the number of muscle fibers in a human is fixed early on in his or her life. Myofibers are regulated by myostatin, a cytokine that is synthesized in muscle cells (and circulates as a hormone later in life). Myostatin suppresses skeletal muscle development.

In adults, increased strength and muscle mass comes about through an increase in the thickness of the individual fibers and increase in the amount of connective tissue, not through an increase in the number of myofibers. Myoblasts release interleukin 4 (IL-4) to attract each other. Muscle fibers, though, are just the building blocks for whole muscles. The precise way in which fibers are arranged into muscle is referred to as architecture. Skeletal muscle is organized to function at both the microscopic and macroscopic level. The functional properties of a whole muscle depend strongly on its architecture.

Understanding muscle architecture is necessary to understand the functional properties of different skeletal muscles. There are three common skeletal muscle arrangements: parallel (longitudinally) arranged, unipennate, multipennate, and circular (Figure 4.34). Parallel muscles have fibers that extend parallel to the muscle force-generating axis (Figure 4.34). Although the fibers extend parallel to the force-generating axis, they never

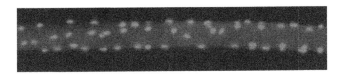

FIGURE 4.33   Fluorescent image of an isolated myofiber. (From Pichavant, C. and Pavlath, G.K., *Skeletal Muscle*, 4, 9, 2014.)

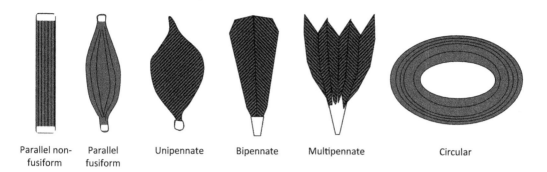

Parallel non-fusiform   Parallel fusiform   Unipennate   Bipennate   Multipennate   Circular

FIGURE 4.34   Different types of skeletal muscle based on the orientation of their fibers.

extend the entire muscle length. Biceps are an example. Unipennate muscles have fibers that are oriented at a single angle relative to the force-generating axis (Figure 4.34). The angle between the fiber and the force-generating axis generally varies from 0° to 30°. The vastus lateralis is an example. Multipennate muscles are composed of fibers that are oriented at several angles relative to the axis of force generation (Figure 4.34). Most muscles fall into this category; the gluteus medius is an example. Circular muscles (sphincters) have fibers that are concentrically arranged around an opening or recess (Figure 4.34). When the muscle contracts the diameter of the opening decreases. Sphincters guard entrances and exits of internal passageways including the digestive and urinary tracts. The orbicularis oris muscle of the mouth is an example.

4.9.2   Skeletal Muscle Internal Arrangement

Skeletal muscle fibers show a pattern of cross banding, they are also called *striated muscle*. The banding is a result of the protein arrangement in the sarcomere, the basic unit of a myofiber (Figure 4.35).[23] The pattern is created by alternating protein bands, the A bands (dark) and the I bands (light). In the center of each A band is a lighter zone called the *H zone*. In the center of each I band is a dark, thin line called the *Z line*. The sarcomere is between two Z lines, the sarcomere is the contractile unit in skeletal muscle.[2,21]

Each sarcomere is composed of two sets of protein filament, myosin and actin (Figure 4.4). These are the principal force-generating components in the sarcomere. Thick myosin filaments are made up of many myosin molecules and are located in the A band. Myosin has a globular head end and a tail section (Figure 4.35). The center part of the filament contains only the tail regions because the molecules are oriented oppositely in either end of the filament in a bipolar arrangement (Figure 4.35). Actin is located primarily in filaments in the I bands but extends into the A bands (Figure 4.35). The thin filaments also contain smaller amounts of two other proteins, troponin and tropomyosin (Figure 4.35). The overlap of the actin and myosin filaments causes the dark coloration of the A bands. The myofilaments are arranged in interdigitating matrices capable of sliding across each other.

To produce force, crossbridges from the myosin, filaments associate with the actin filament. Then they rotate slightly to pull the filaments across each other (similar to the oars of a rowboat pull across the water). The bipolar arrangement of the myosin molecules causes the action of the crossbridges to draw the thin filaments inward from both

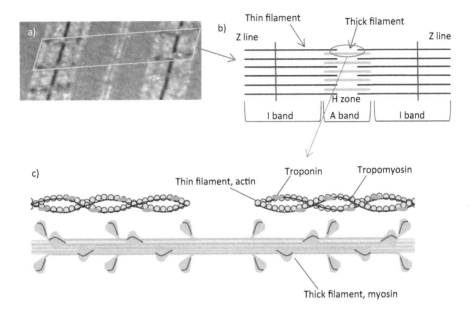

FIGURE 4.35 Images of the sarcomere in skeletal muscle, (a) SEM image of the sarcomeres, (From Tsai, F-C., et al., *J. Neurotrauma.*, 27, 1509–1516, 2010.) (b) a diagram of a sarcomere, close up image of a thick filament and thin filament in a sarcomere.

directions. The globular myosin heads (on thick filaments) have binding sites for the actin molecules (on the thin filaments) and ATP.

Calcium ions (Ca^{2+}) link action potentials in a muscle fiber to contraction. In resting muscle fibers, Ca^{2+} is stored in the endoplasmic (sarcoplasmic) reticulum. Along the plasma membrane (sarcolemma) of the muscle fiber are inpockets of the membrane that form the trans-tubules of the "T system" (Figure 4.36). These tubules plunge repeatedly into the interior of the fiber near the calcium-filled sacs of the sarcoplasmic reticulum (Figure 4.36). The sarcoplasmic reticulums are large and work their way throughout the length and circumference of each myofiber (Figure 4.36). Each action potential created at the neuromuscular junction sweeps quickly along the sarcolemma and is carried into the T system. The arrival of the action potential at the ends of the T system triggers the release

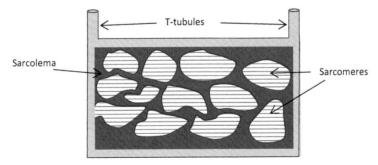

FIGURE 4.36 A two-dimensional representation of the t-tubules (pink) and sarcolemma (red) in skeletal muscle. The sarcolemma come into contact with the sarcomeres (blue stripes) in the myofibers to release calcium throughout the muscle.

of Ca^{2+}. The Ca^{2+} diffuses among the thick and thin filaments where it binds to troponin on the thin filaments. This turns on the interaction between actin and myosin and the sarcomere contracts. Because of the speed of the action potential (milliseconds), the action potential arrives virtually simultaneously at the ends of all the tubules of the T system, ensuring that all sarcomeres contract in unison. When the process is over, the calcium is pumped back into the sarcoplasmic reticulum using a Ca^{2+} ATPase.

Activation of the muscle fiber causes the myosin heads to bind to actin. A change occurs that draws the thin filament a short distance (~10 nm) past the thick filament. Then the linkages break (for which ATP is needed) and reform farther along the thin filament to repeat the process. As a result, the filaments are pulled past each other in a ratchet-like action.

As a muscle contracts, the Z lines come closer together and the width of the I bands and H zones decrease. There no change in the width of the A band. Conversely, as a muscle is stretched, the width of the I bands and H zones increases, but there is no change in the width of the A band. The shortening of the sarcomeres in a myofibril shortens the myofibril and the muscle fiber that it belongs to. Muscle force is proportional to physiologic cross-sectional area (PCSA), and muscle velocity is proportional to muscle fiber length. PCSA is the sum of the areas of each fiber in the muscle.

There are two different types of muscle fiber in most skeletal muscles, Type I and Type II fibers. Type I fibers have lots of mitochondria and depend on cellular respiration for ATP production. They are rich in myoglobin, which gives them a reddish color, and resistant to fatigue. They are activated by small-diameter, thus slow-conducting, motor neurons and are known as "slow-twitch" fibers. These slow-twitch fibers are the main muscles used for tone and posture.

Type II fibers have far fewer mitochondria than Type I fibers and are rich in glycogen. They depend on glycolysis for ATP production and fatigue easily. Type II fibers are low in myoglobin, which gives them a whitish color. These fibers are activated by fast conducting, large-diameter motor neurons, so they are known as "fast-twitch" fibers. Fast-twitch fibers are dominant in muscles used for rapid movement.

Most skeletal muscles contain some mixture of Type I and Type II fibers, but a single motor unit always contains one type or the other, never both. The ratio of Type I and Type II fibers can be changed by endurance training (producing more Type I fibers).

4.9.3 Cardiac Muscle

Cardiac muscle is striated like skeletal muscle. Each cell contains sarcomeres with sliding filaments of actin and myosin. Unlike skeletal muscle, cardiac muscle is made up of single cells with a single nucleus (Figure 4.37).[24] The cells are connected end-to-end, and to a lesser extent, side-by-side. Some of the cells may branch so that one end connects to two other cells. At the connections between cells, there is a specialized structure called the *intercalated disc* (Figure 4.37).[24] Intercalated discs are areas of extremely close contact where there is no intercellular space. These discs have many projections into each cell which form an undulating double membrane that separates the adjacent cells. There are three types of membrane junctions exist within an intercalated disc, the fascia adherens, macula adherens, and gap junctions.

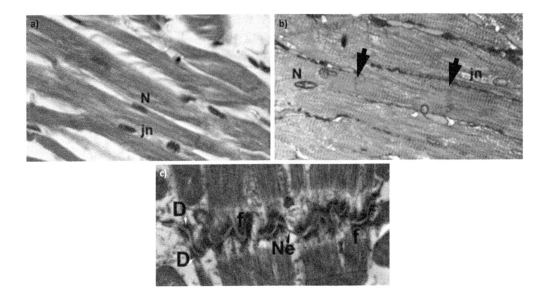

FIGURE 4.37 Pictures of cardiac myoblasts. (a) shows that cardiac muscle is made up of many connected single cells with one nucleus (N and jn); (b) shows the presence of striations as a result of sarcomeres, single nuclei (N and jn), and the presence of intercolated discs (arrows); and (c) shows the intercalated disc, desmosomes (D), fasciae adherens (f), and gap junctions (Ne). (From El-Deeb, M.E.E. and Abd-El-Hafez, A.A.A., *J. Microsc. Ultrastruct.*, 3, 120–136, 2015.[24])

Fascia adherens are the anchoring sites for actin; they also connect to the closest sarcomere. Desmosomes prevent separation of cells during contraction by binding the intermediate filaments joining the cells together. This creates a strong mechanical connection between cells. They are also called a *macula adherens*. These strong junctions enable the heart to contract forcefully without ripping the fibers apart. Gap junctions allow action potentials to spread between cardiac cells by allowing ions to pass between cells; these ions produce the depolarization of the heart muscle, which causes the action potential. The gap junctions provide a close electrical connection between cells. Unlike skeletal muscle, the action potential that triggers the heartbeat is generated within the heart itself. The action potential that drives contraction of the heart passes from fiber to fiber through gap junctions.

4.9.4 Smooth Muscle

Smooth muscle is made of single, spindle-shaped cells; its name comes from the fact that there are no visible striations. Although striations are not visible each smooth muscle cell contains thick (myosin) and thin (actin) filaments that slide against each other to produce contraction of the cell. The thick and thin filaments are anchored near the plasma membrane using intermediate filaments (Figure 4.38). When they contract, they change the shape of the smooth muscle cells, making them shorter and thicker (Figure 4.38). Smooth muscle is used to change the diameters of hollow tissues and organs like blood vessels, bladder, intestines, and uterus.

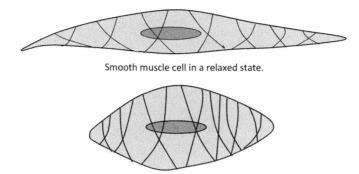

Smooth muscle cell in a relaxed state.

Smooth muscle in a contracted state.

FIGURE 4.38   Smooth muscle cells in a relaxed state and a contracted state.

4.10 IMPORTANCE TO TISSUE ENGINEERING

Knowledge of tissue composition and function is extremely important in tissue engineering. Every tissue is different. Each tissue serves a different purpose, so they have different mechanical properties, densities, conductivities, etc. Each tissue is designed to support a selected cell type so that it can thrive in that particular environment. Having in-depth knowledge of the tissue that you are replacing or regenerating is valuable for the selection of materials to be used in the replacement of the structure of the replacement, fibrous, hydrogel, ceramic, etc. Being informed about the original tissue can give the engineer the necessary information to provide the optimal environment for the cell type typically found in the tissue that you are replacing. This will lead to a restoration of biological activity and regeneration of new tissue. Knowledge of the mechanical properties will prevent the implanted device from being crushed, torn apart, or tearing away from surrounding tissue. The strength of a material can also positively or negatively affect the behavior of the cells seeded on it. So matching the mechanical properties of the native tissue will aid in restoring biological activity of the cells.

4.11 QUESTIONS

1. What is the difference between an aligned matrix and an alignable matrix?

2. What does elastin do in arterial blood vessels?

3. Describe the different structures in long bones.

4. Describe the structural differences among skeletal muscle, cardiac muscle, and smooth muscle.

5. Describe how neurons regenerate? Can a neuron proliferate (split and produce daughter cells)?

6. Name four types of skeletal muscle and describe them.

7. How are astrocytes and oligodendrocytes similar? How are they different?

8. What are the differences between arterial vessels and venous vessels?

9. What other tissues are housed in bone?

10. Are tendons and muscles easily separated? Why or why not?

REFERENCES

1. Berne RM, Levy MN, Koeppen BM, Stanton BA (Eds.). Physiology. 4th ed. St/Louis, MO: Mosby; 1998.
2. Widmaier EP, Raff H, Strang KT (Eds.). *Vander's Human Physiology: The Mechanisms of Body Function*. 12th ed. Columbus, OH: McGraw-Hill Education; 2010.
3. Rhoades R, Pflanzer R (Eds.). *Human Physiology*. 3rd ed. Orlando, FL: Saunders College Publishing; 1989.
4. Mow VC, Hayes WC (Eds.) *Basic Orthopaedic Biomechanics*. 2nd ed. Philadelphia, PA: Lippincott-Raven; 1997.
5. Cowin SC, Doty SB. *Tissue Mechanics*. New York: Springer; 2007.
6. Wikimedia Foundation I. Osteon: Wikimedia Foundation; 2018. Available from: https://en.wikipedia.org/wiki/Osteon.
7. Fu Q, Saiz E et al. Bioactive glass scaffolds for bone tissue engineering: state of the art and future perspectives. *Materials Science & Engineering C, Materials for Biological Applications*. 2011 31(7):1245–1256.
8. Ku L, DL W et al. *Tissue Engineering And Biodegradable Equivalents, Scientific And Clinical Applications*. New York: Marcel Dekker; 2002.
9. Liu X, Rahaman MN et al. Mechanical properties of bioactive glass (13–93) scaffolds fabricated by robotic deposition for structural bone repair. *Acta Biomaterialia*. 2013 9(6):7025–7034.
10. Kastelic J, Galeski A et al. The multicomposite structure of tendon. *Connective Tissue Research*. 1978 6(1):11–23.
11. McBridge DJ. Hind limb extensor tendon development in the chick: A light and transmission electron microscopic study. Newark, NJ: Rutgers University; 1984.
12. Bartel DL, Davy DT et al. *Orthopaedic Biomechanics: Mechanics and Design in Musculoskeletal Systems*. Upper Saddle River, NJ: Pearson/Prentice Hall; 2006.
13. Mow VC, Ratcliffe A. Structure and function of articular cartilage and meniscus. In: Mow VC, Hayes WC (Eds.). *Basic Orthopaedic Biomechanics*. 2nd ed. Philadelphia, PA: Lippincott Raven Publishers; 1997. pp. 113–177.
14. Tsuchida AI, Beekhuizen M et al. Cytokine profiles in the joint depend on pathology, but are different between synovial fluid, cartilage tissue and cultured chondrocytes. *Arthritis Research & Therapy*. 2014 16(5):441.
15. Wilson W, Driessen NJ et al. Prediction of collagen orientation in articular cartilage by a collagen remodeling algorithm. *Osteoarthritis and Cartilage*. 2006 14(11):1196–1202.
16. Karim A, Amin AK et al. The clustering and morphology of chondrocytes in normal and mildly degenerate human femoral head cartilage studied by confocal laser scanning microscopy. *Journal of Anatomy*. 2018 232(4):686–698.
17. King D. Elastic cartilage 2009 [updated December 16, 2009]. Available from: http://www.siumed.edu/~dking2/ssb/NM011b.htm.
18. Auffarth A, Resch H et al. Cartilage morphological and histological findings after reconstruction of the glenoid with an iliac crest bone graft. *American Journal of Sports Medicine*. 2018 46(5):1039–1045.
19. Purves D, Augustine GJ, Fitzpatrick D, Hall WC, Lamantia A-S, Mcnamara JO et al. (Eds.). *Neuroscience*. 3rd ed. Sunderland, MA: Sinauer Associates; 2004.

20. American Association of Neurological Surgeons. Anatomy of the brain: American association of neurological surgeons; 2018. Available from: http://www.aans.org/Patients/Neurosurgical-Conditions-and-Treatments/Anatomy-of-the-Brain.
21. Berne RM, Levy MN, Koeppen BM, Stanton BA (Eds.). *Physiology*. Fourth ed. St/Louis, MO: Mosby; 1998.
22. Pichavant C, Pavlath GK. Incidence and severity of myofiber branching with regeneration and aging. *Skeletal Muscle*. 2014 4:9.
23. Tsai F-C, Hsieh M-S et al. Comparison between neurectomy and botulinum toxin A injection for denervated skeletal muscle. *Journal of Neurotrauma*. 2010 27(8):1509–1516.
24. El-Deeb MEE, Abd-El-Hafez AAA. Can vitamin C affect the $KBrO_3$ induced oxidative stress on left ventricular myocardium of adult male albino rats? A histological and immunohistochemical study. *Journal of Microscopy and Ultrastructure*. 2015 3(3):120–136.

Materials for Tissue Engineering

5.1 INTRODUCTION

To create scaffolds that have the appropriate mechanical and biological properties, researchers have used a wide variety of materials. Synthetic polymers are frequently used because they allow the researcher to have control over the properties of the material, including strength, hydrophilicity, and charge. Natural materials are used because of their inherent bioactivity and biocompatibility. In some cases, decellularized tissues are used because they contain a host of natural materials with biocompatibility and bioactivity with specific mechanical strength and a specific architecture.

5.2 SYNTHETIC POLYMERS

Polymers represent a versatile class of biomaterial that has been extensively investigated. They have flexibility in synthesis and in modification. We can use this flexibility to match the properties of various tissues or organs in the body. The first synthetic polymeric biomaterials were used in the 1940s, with the introduction of poly(methyl methacrylate) (PMMA), used as a corneal implant (Figure 5.1). This sparked the use of many other "off-the-shelf" polymers for tissue replacement, such as hip joint replacements, intraocular lenses, and blood-contacting devices. However, the long-term biocompatibility of many of these materials was a serious concern. During the latter half of the twentieth century, materials scientists began attempts to engineer novel polymeric materials or modify existing polymers to exhibit biocompatibility, provide adequate mechanical properties, and be suitable for specific biomedical applications. To select the correct polymer for the correct application researchers are concerned with strength, transition temperatures, and stability (degradability).

The strength of a polymeric material depends on its chemistry. Specifically, characteristics such as the length and size of polymer chains, degree of crystallinity, transition temperatures, and chemistry of the side groups all affect a polymer's strength.

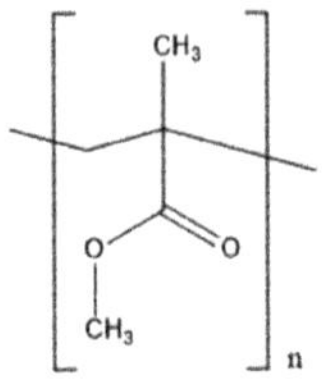

FIGURE 5.1   Structure of poly(methyl methacrylate) (PMMA).

Polymer chain length effects strength by increasing the number of potential interactions with nearby chains. The longer the chain, the more chain-to-chain interactions (bonding or entanglements) there are, resulting in greater strength. Larger side groups can lead to greater entanglements or more inhibitions to sliding of polymer chains by one another. Large side groups can also cause more interactions with the backbone or side groups of neighboring chains.

The degree of crystallinity is a measure of polymer chain organization. As the level of organization between neighboring polymer chains increases, a polymer becomes more crystalline. As the organization between the chains decreases, the polymer becomes more amorphous. The higher the degree of crystallinity, the more polymer chains line up alongside one another, which increases the number of chain-to-chain interactions, which then increases polymer strength (Figure 5.2). Crystallinity is affected by the size of side groups, the distribution of side groups (random or regular), and nature of side groups (charged, aromatic, etc.). Polymer crystallinity can be increased by cooling polymers slowly and applying tension during processing. No polymer is 100% crystalline; there will always be amorphous sections.

The chemistry of the polymer also plays a role in its strength. The ability to form bonds (hydrogen, ionic, crosslinks) with neighboring chains increases strength. As the number of potential bonding sites increases, the polymer strength increases.

The mechanical properties of polymers can be affected by heating. The addition of heat gives energy to the polymer chains, which increases their mobility. At specific temperatures, the chains become so mobile that they cause a change in the overall polymer mechanical properties; these are transition temperatures. These changes occur at T_g, the glass transition temperature, and T_m, the melting temperature (Figure 5.3). All polymers have a T_g and T_m. Crystalline polymers have a crystalline melting point, going from a crystalline solid to a melt. At T_g, the polymer goes from a rubber to a glass, from flexible to stiff. This happens in amorphous polymers. At T_m, the polymer goes from a solid to a melt. As a melt, the polymer flows. So for flexible tissues, you want an amorphous polymer with a T_g that is lower than room or body temp. For hard tissues you want a crystalline polymer, which means you want a T_g and T_m that give you the properties that you need at body temperature (Figure 5.3).

Degradability is a huge issue in tissue engineering. As we look to repair damaged tissue through more regenerative approaches, there is a greater need for structures that will not remain in the body permanently. Optimally researchers want the polymer to degrade and be cleared from the body while cells grow new tissue *in vivo*. There are two general types of

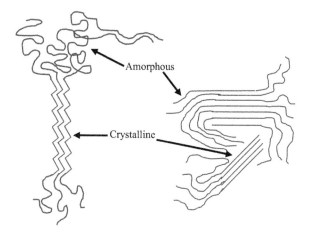

FIGURE 5.2   Two schematics of polymers with crystalline and amorphous structures.

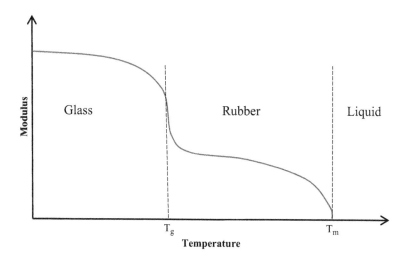

FIGURE 5.3   Plot of temperature vs. modulus displaying the glass transition temperature (T_g) and melting temperature (T_m).

degradation that we see in biomaterials, hydrolytic and enzymatic. Hydrolytic degradation is caused by exposure to water. Enzymatic degradation depends on cells producing enzymes to break down the polymer. Therefore, polymers that degrade enzymatically typically have linkages based on amine groups (NH_2). The vast majority of synthetic polymers used in tissue engineering degrade hydrolytically. Hydrolytically degradable polymers can degrade by two different mechanisms, bulk and surface (Figure 5.4). During bulk degradation, the water penetrates the thickness of a polymeric device exposing a large amount of the volume to water. In this model, material is lost from the entire polymer volume at the same time because of water penetrating the bulk. The rate of degradation of these polymers depends on the extent of water accessibility to the matrix rather than the intrinsic rate of ester cleavage. The water accessibility to the matrix depends on several factors: the hydrophobicity or hydrophilicity of the polymer, the crystallinity of the polymer, and the dimensions of the sample. In surface

Bulk degradation over time

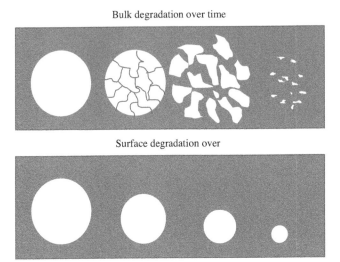

Surface degradation over

FIGURE 5.4 A schematic depicting bulk and surface degradation.

degradation, water cannot penetrate the volume of the device, therefore only the surface is accessible for degradation. As you can imagine if we need to maintain device strength or have the device remain for longer periods of time, surface degradation is preferred. In this case, you can enhance the rate of degradation by increasing the surface area of the object. Thin sheets are examples of shapes with high surface area, whereas spheres have lower surface area. In the thin sheet, more of the polymer is exposed to the surroundings, whereas in the sphere, more of the polymer is within the shape, not exposed to the surroundings (Figure 5.5).

5.2.1 Types of Polymers

The trend in biomedical engineering is moving toward materials with bioactivity, biocompatibility, and biodegradability. Degradation prevents stress shielding of new tissue, and, eventually, the polymer disappears and new tissue is left. The transient existence of materials is highly preferred for *in vivo* applications such as implantable drug-delivery systems and conduits for guiding or remodeling damaged tissues. With biostable polymers, in most cases, a second surgical procedure must be performed to remove the implant to overcome

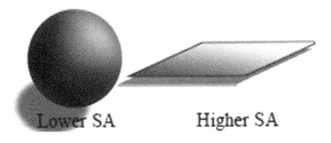

FIGURE 5.5 Examples of structures with high and low surface area (SA).

long-term biocompatibility issues. Biodegradable polymers are those which degrade *in vitro* and *in vivo*. They degrade into normal metabolites of the body and into products that can be completely eliminated from the body with or without further metabolic transformations. The basic criteria of selection of a biodegradable polymer as a biomaterial are that its degradation products should be nontoxic. The rate of degradation and mechanical properties of the material should match the intended application. In drug-delivery systems, fine-tuning of drug release kinetics is possible by varying the degradation rate of the matrix polymer. With synthetic polymers, it is possible to develop polymers with a wide spectrum of properties with excellent reproducibility. Fine-tuning of the degradation rate of these polymers is feasible by varying their structure.

5.2.1.1 Aliphatic Polyesters

Aliphatic polyesters, Figure 5.6, can be considered representatives of synthetic biodegradable polymers. The low melting points, low hydrolytic stability, and low molecular weights of the polymers initially obtained severely limited their application. At the same time, the high hydrolytic instability of these polymers resulted in a multitude of applications for this polymer class in the biomedical field starting with absorbable sutures in the 1960s. The commonly used monomers for aliphatic polyester synthesis for biomedical applications are lactide, glycolide, and caprolactone. Poly(glycolic acid) (PGA) was one of the initially investigated biodegradable polyesters for biomedical applications. It is a highly crystalline polymer with a melting point greater than 200°C and T_g of 35°C–40°C. Because of its high crystallinity, PGA shows high tensile strength and modulus, but very low solubility in common organic solvents. The initial applications of PGA were directed toward developing biodegradable sutures and the first biodegradable synthetic. PGA was also investigated as a material for the development of internal bone fixation devices. The high degradation rate of the polymer and low solubility coupled with the accumulation of acidic degradation products, which can lead to inflammatory reactions, limits its application in the biomedical field (Figures 5.7 and 5.8).

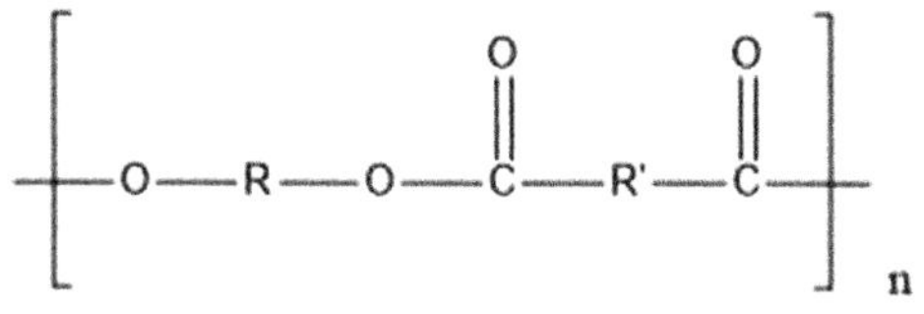

FIGURE 5.6   Structure of a generic polyester.

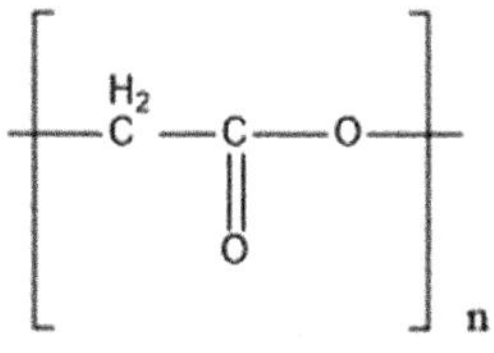

FIGURE 5.7   Structure of polyglycolic acid (PGA).

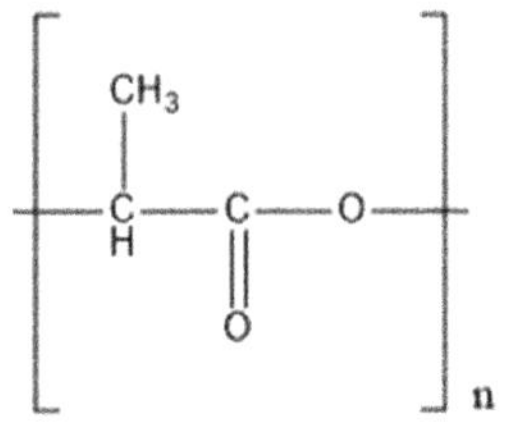

FIGURE 5.8 Structure of polactic acid (PLA).

Lactide is a chiral molecule, the polymer exists as three isomers: L-lactide, D-lactide, and meso-lactide. There are four different types of poly(lactic acid) (PLA): Poly(L-lactic acid), poly(D-lactic acid), poly(DL-lactic acid), and meso-poly(lactic acid). Poly(L-lactic acid) and poly(DL-lactic acid) have been extensively investigated as biomaterials. Poly(L-lactic acid) (PLLA) is semi crystalline, where the degree of crystallinity depends on the molecular weight and processing parameters. It has a high modulus and strength, and a melting point of around 170°C, and a T_g of about 60°C–65°C. PDLLA is an amorphous polymer caused by the random distribution of the two isomeric forms along the polymer chain. It has a T_g of about 55°C–60°C. PLA has been extensively investigated as a bone fixative, with a low degradation rate, better processability, and mechanical properties (Figure 5.8).

Poly(caprolactone), Figure 5.9, is a semi crystalline polyester. Its melting temperature is around 55°C–60°C and has a T_g of –60°C. It can be obtained from cheap starting material (caprolactone), has high solubility in organic solvents, a low melting point, and T_g, and the ability to form blends with a variety of polymers. Because of its low degradation rate, PCL has been investigated as a material for the long-term controlled delivery of drugs. A long-term contraceptive device, Capronor, based on PCL has already been placed on the market. You can fine-tune properties by copolymerizing the respective monomers. Copolymers of PLA and PGA (PLAGA) have been extensively investigated, including suture, bone pins, stents, drug-delivery devices, and scaffolds for tissue engineering (Figure 5.10).

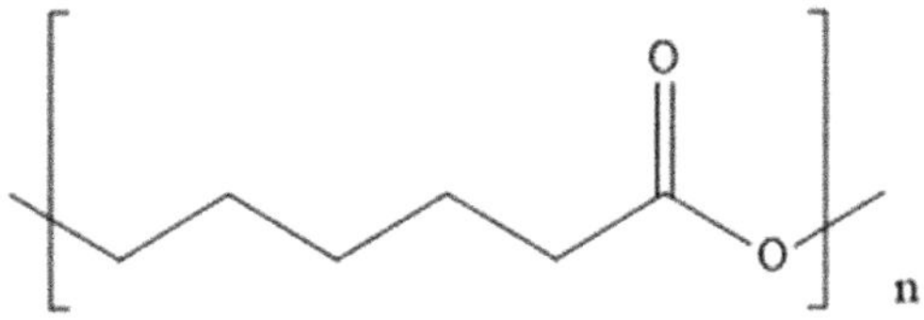

FIGURE 5.9 Structure of polycaprolactone (PCL).

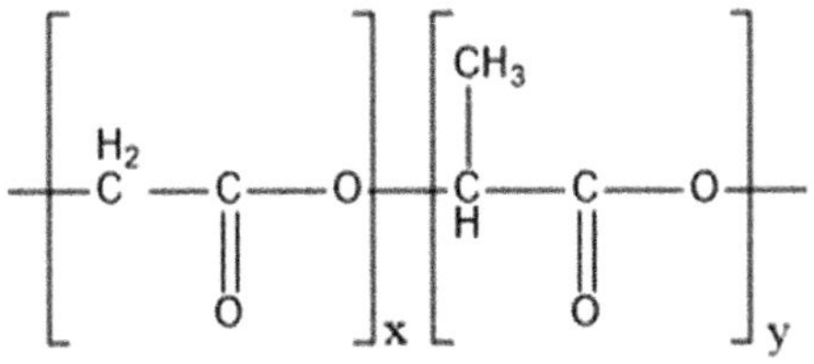

FIGURE 5.10 Copolymer of PLA and PGA. PLAGA.

The mechanical and degradation properties of these polymers can be tailored depending on the copolymer ratios. The aliphatic polyesters undergo bulk degradation. The material is lost from the entire polymer volume at the same time because of water penetrating the bulk. The rate of degradation of these polymers depends on the extent of water accessibility to the matrix rather than the intrinsic rate of ester cleavage. The water accessibility to the matrix depends on several factors: the hydrophobicity or hydrophilicity of the polymer, the crystallinity of the polymer, and the dimensions of the sample.

5.2.1.2 Polyanhydrides

Polyanhydrides form another class of surface-eroding polymers. They have been extensively studied solely for biomedical applications. They are very hydrolytically unstable. The low hydrolytic stability and low molecular weight of many of these polymers barred them from any industrial application. In 1980 Langer et al. proposed them as ideal candidates for drug-delivery applications. Polyanhydrides have a highly hydrophobic backbone and a highly hydrolytically sensitive anhydride bond. This matrix hydrophobicity prevents water penetration into the matrix, so the degradation and erosion of the polymer are essentially confined to the surface. Aliphatic homopolymers such as poly(sebacic anhydride) (PSA) are highly crystalline and have very high degradation rates that severely limit their application. Aromatic polyanhydrides, on the other hand, have very high hydrolytic stability and very high melting points, which make them difficult to process. Moreover, it has been established that the anhydride bonds between aliphatic carboxylic acids degrade faster than those of aromatic carboxylic acids. The degradation rate of polyanhydrides is a function of the polymer structure as well as the type of monomers used. This led to the development of various aliphatic-aromatic polyanhydrides. Their properties can be tailored by varying the ratios of the two monomers. The most extensively investigated of these polymers is poly[(carboxy phenoxy)propanesebacic acid] (PCPP-SA). Recently, the FDA has approved PCPP-SA as a delivery matrix for the controlled delivery of the chemotherapeutic agent BCNU to treat brain cancer under the trade name Gliadel.

5.2.1.3 Poly(amino acids)

Synthetic poly(amino acids), Figure 5.11, have been investigated for various biomedical applications because of their structural similarity with naturally occurring proteins. The high crystallinity, low degradation rate, unfavorable mechanical properties, and immunogenicity of these polymers has limited their biomedical applications. Therefore, several different amino acid derived polymers have been developed. The amino acid derived

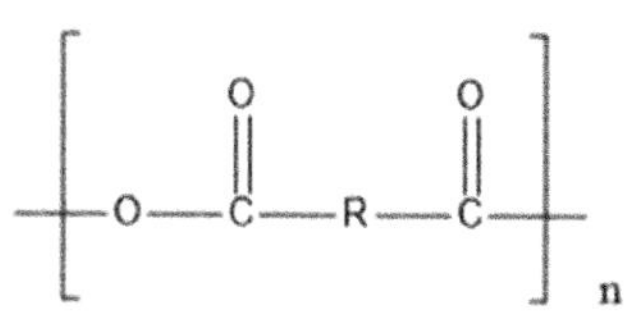

FIGURE 5.11 Structure of a generic polyanhydride.

polymers were synthesized by grafting amino acids on synthetic polymers, copolymerizing amino acids with other monomers, synthesizing block copolymers having amino acid sequences and poly(ethylene glycol), and developing pseudo poly(amino acids) where the amino acid monomers are linked by non-amide bonds such as ester, carbonate, or imino carbonate bonds. One of the more extensively studied pseudo amino acid polymer is the tyrosine-derived pseudo poly(amino acid). Tyrosine is a naturally occurring aromatic amino acid that can give good mechanical properties to the corresponding polymers. The physicochemical properties of these polymers can be altered by varying the pendant alkyl ester chain. These polymers are hydrophobic and amorphous with T_g less than 100°C and decomposition temperatures around 300°C. The final degradation products of the polymer are tyrosine and the diols used to esterify the side chain. Because of the slow degradation rate of these polymers, tyrosine carbonates (desaminotyrosyl-tyrosine alkyl esters, DTH), have been investigated as matrices for the long-term delivery of drugs. Poly(DTH-carbonates) is osteocompatible. Poly(imino carbonates) based on natural amino acid L-tyrosine or its derivatives have been studied as amorphous, biodegradable polymers. They have high mechanical strength and stiffness. Poly(DTH-imino carbonate) has been found to be a promising candidate for transient medical applications because of its better degradability, low processing temperature, high mechanical strength, and better processability.

5.2.1.4 Polyphosphazenes

All of the synthetic biodegradable polymers we have discussed are organic polymers (i.e., carbon in the backbone). Inorganic polymers have backbones that contain atoms other than carbon, nitrogen, or oxygen. This gives these polymers unique properties. Polyphosphazenes are in this class of polymers. Polyphosphazenes form a versatile class of inorganic polymers as a result of their synthetic flexibility and high adaptability for applications. These are linear, high molecular-weight polymers with an inorganic backbone of alternating phosphorus and nitrogen atoms. Each phosphorus atom bears two organic side groups. The unique feature of polyphosphazenes is that the side groups play a crucial role in determining their physical properties. This gives us the opportunity to create a large number of polymers from a basic polyphosphazene. The macromolecular substitution route allows for the introduction of two or more different side groups on a basic polyphosphazene (such as polydichlorophosphazene) through simultaneous or sequential substitution, which results in polymers with a wide spectrum of properties. The phosphorus-nitrogen backbone can be rendered hydrolytically unstable when substituted with appropriate organic side groups on the phosphorus atoms. Adding organic side groups such as amino acid esters, amines, imidazole, or alkoxide groups impart degradability to polyphosphazenes (Figure 5.12).

The degradation products of these polymers were found to be neutral and nontoxic (phosphates, ammonia, and the corresponding side groups). The degradation rate of the polymers can be fine-tuned by incorporating fewer or more highly hydrolytically sensitive groups. The degradation rate of these polymers depends on the nature of the side groups, the ratio of the side groups, the pH of the surrounding medium, temperature,

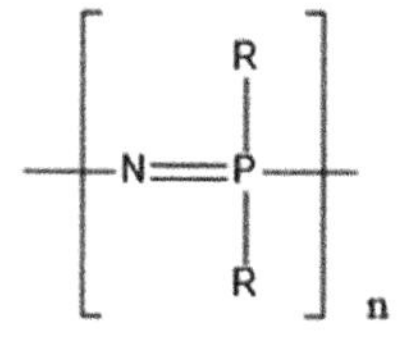

FIGURE 5.12   Structure of a generic polyphosphazene.

and solubility of the degradation products. The synthetic versatility of polyphosphazenes makes it possible to design novel polymers with a desired degradation profile. This can be translated into designing drug release systems based primarily on diffusion, erosion, or a mixture of erosion and diffusion. Biodegradable polyphosphazenes are now being extensively investigated as matrices for drug-delivery applications, particularly protein delivery. The biocompatibility of these polymers makes them candidates for tissue engineering. Several biodegradable polyphosphazenes are under investigation for bone and neural tissue engineering applications. The presence of phosphorus in polyphosphazenes provides active sites to which drug molecules can be attached, enabling the development of targeted delivery systems.

5.3 BIOMACROMOLECULES

When looking to create tissue-engineered constructs one common place to look for materials is nature. After all, we are made from some of these materials and others we have interacted with for decades (in some cases even a millennia). In addition, because they are not petroleum based, these materials allow us to work in a sustainable way. Nature presents us with numerous materials from numerous sources. Animal and human tissues are excellent resources for tissue engineers. These materials have known biocompatibility and bioactivity. We can extract biopolymers from tissues and purify them for later use. We can extract the mineral from ground bone or even precipitate forms of calcium phosphate in the laboratory for use in implantable devices. Their known characteristics, biocompatibility, and bioactivity make then highly sought after. Unfortunately, there may be differences in quality and even properties when comparing one batch of material derived from tissue to another. In addition, currently accepted modes of sterilization can denature proteins, this could weaken the device before it is implanted. Biomacromolecules such as cellulose are found in plants and are produced by bacteria. As the most abundant biomaterial on the planet cellulose is relatively inexpensive. Unfortunately, it cannot be degraded in the human body, so the material must be pretreated before implantation. In this chapter we will describe these materials and give some examples of their use. In some cases, we will refer back to our previous chapter on tissues to provide more in-depth discussions.

Biomacromolecules (polysaccharides and proteins) have excellent biocompatibility, unique mechanical properties, closely mimic native cellular environments, and are biodegradable by an enzymatic or hydrolytic mechanism. They also have a risk of viral infection, antigenicity, unstable material supply, and batch-to-batch variation in properties. Many of the materials listed in this section have been explained in more depth in the chapter on tissues.

5.3.1 Polysaccharides

Polysaccharides are high molecular-weight polymers having one or more monosaccharide repeating units. The advantages associated with polysaccharides include widespread availability, cost effectiveness, and a wide range of properties and structures. Polysaccharides can also be easily modified because of the presence of reactive functional groups along the polymer chain. Their biodegradability, biocompatibility, water solubility, and ability to form hydrogels make them excellent candidates for tissue engineering and drug-delivery applications.

5.3.1.1 Polysaccharides: Hyaluronic Acid

Hyaluronic acid is a naturally occurring linear anionic polysaccharide consisting of repeating disaccharide units, Figure 5.13. It is an important component of articular cartilage and is widely distributed in the connective tissue as well as vitreous and synovial fluids of mammals. The polymer is water soluble, forming very viscous solutions. Hyaluronic acid possesses several properties that make it an ideal candidate for wound dressing applications. It can act as a scavenger for free radicals in wounds, controlling inflammation. It can interact with a variety of biomolecules, is a bacteriostat, and can be recognized by receptors on a variety of cells associated with tissue repair. Cross-linked hyaluronic acid gels or hyaluronic acid derivatives such as ethyl/benzyl (HYAFF) esters have been investigated for wound-dressing applications. The rate of degradation and the solubility of the hyaluronic acid can be controlled by changing the extent of esterification. These derivatives can be fabricated into a variety of shapes such as membranes, fibers, sponges, and microspheres. High molecular-weight viscoelastic hyaluronic solutions (AMVISC and AMVISC PLUS) are used to protect delicate tissue in the eye during cataract extraction, corneal transplantation, and glaucoma surgery. Hyaluronic acid can act as a vitreous substitute during retina reattachment surgery. Injectable formulations of hyaluronic acid (SYNVISC, ORTHOVISC) have been developed to relieve pain and improve joint mobility in patients suffering from osteoarthritis.

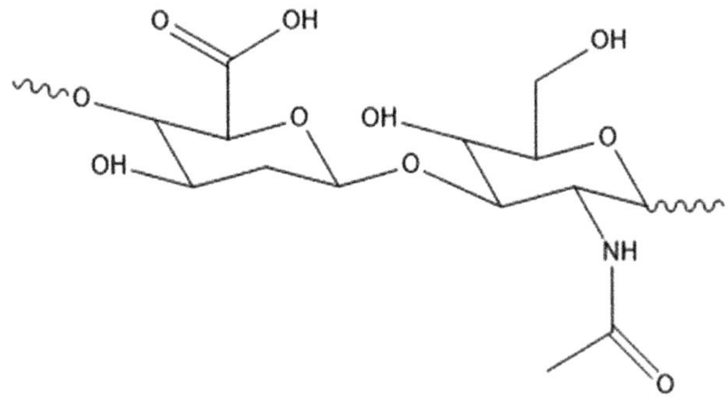

FIGURE 5.13   Structure of hyaluronic acid.

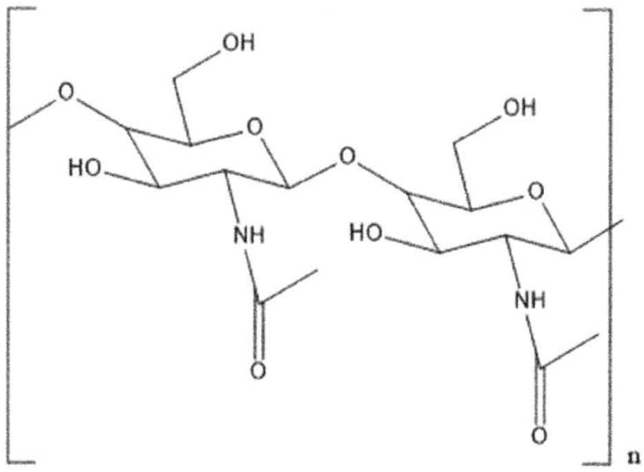

FIGURE 5.14   Chitin structure.

5.3.1.2 Polysaccharides: Chitin and Chitosan

Chitin is a naturally occurring polysaccharide that forms the outer shell of crustaceans, insect exoskeletons, and fungal cell walls, Figure 5.14. It is the second most abundant natural polymer, cellulose being the first. The N-acetyl glucosamino groups in chitin show structural similarity to hyaluronic acid, which has very high wound healing potential. Chitin fibers, mats, sponges, and membranes have been investigated as wound dressing materials.

Chitosan is completely soluble in aqueous solutions with pH lower than 5.0. It undergoes biodegradation *in vivo* enzymatically by lysozymes to nontoxic products. The rate of degradation of chitosan depends inversely on the degree of acetylation and crystallinity of the polymer. Acetyl groups are removed to make chitin into soluble chitosan (Figures 5.15 and 5.16). Chitosan has been investigated as a wound and burn dressing material. It has

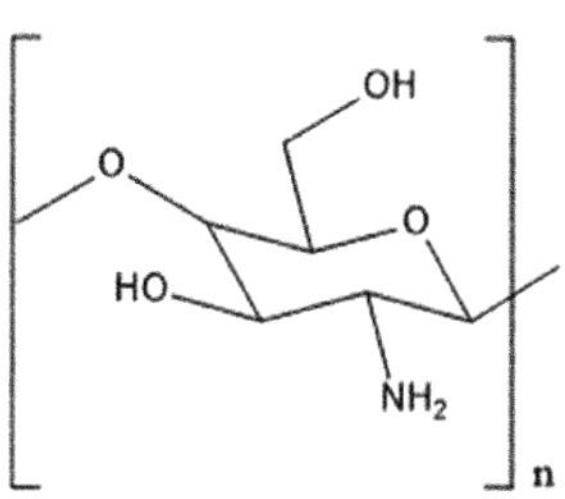

FIGURE 5.15   Chitosan structure.

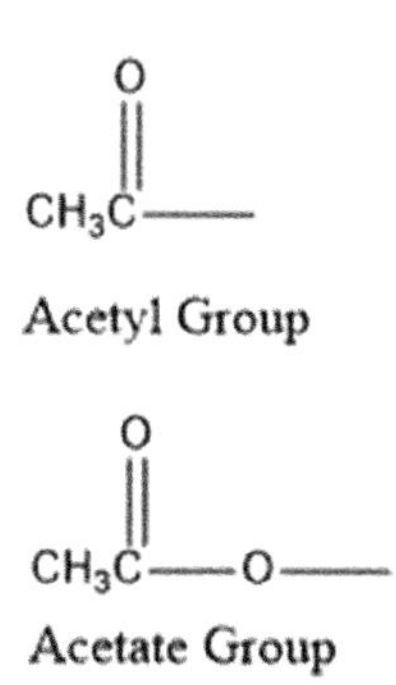

FIGURE 5.16   The difference between an acetyl and acetate group.

easy applicability, oxygen permeability, water absorptivity, haemostatic property, and the ability to induce interleukin-8 from fibroblasts, which is involved in the migration of fibroblasts and endothelial cells. Cross-linked chitosan hydrogel matrices form attractive materials for drug-delivery applications. The rate of drug release can be controlled by varying the cross-linking density. Chitosan is also used to form porous scaffolds for tissue engineering. Chitosan is known to support osteoblast proliferation and phenotype expression.

5.3.1.3 Polysaccharides: Cellulose

Cellulose is the most abundant biopolymer on Earth. It is the major component of plant biomass and is also seen in microbial extracellular polymers. Plant-derived cellulose plays a role in plant structure. Bacterial cellulose (BC) is a primary metabolism and is mainly a protective coating. Chains of BC aggregate to form subfibrils approx. 1.5-nm wide. Subfibrils are crystallized into microfibrils, then bundles, then ribbons. Macroscopic morphology of BC depends on culture conditions. In static conditions, bacteria form mats at the oxygen-rich air-liquid interface. Its ability to grow on surfaces allows BC to form complex shapes easily. It can form a wide variety of shapes for tissue replacement because its surface can be modified to increase biocompatibility, and it can be coated with fibrin, treated to create charged groups for mineralization. BC is biocompatible, but not degradable. BC is created in dense mats, so this can limit cellular infiltration. Usually BC is laid down randomly, but recent work has shown that electric fields can be used to guide that bacteria and create organized BC scaffolds (Figure 5.17).

5.3.2 Proteins

As noted in a previous chapter, proteins are high molecular weight polymers having amino acid repeating units where the amino acids are joined together by characteristic peptide

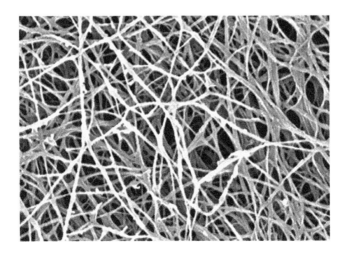

FIGURE 5.17 Electromicrograph of bacterial cellulose.

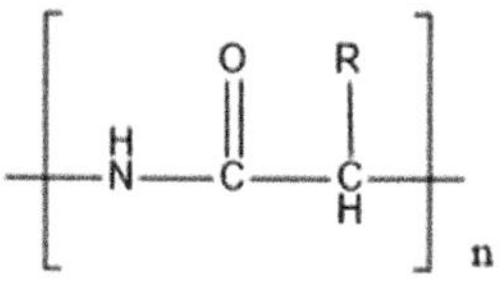

FIGURE 5.18   Generic protein structure.

linkages. These materials have been investigated for various applications such as sutures, hemostatic agents, scaffolds for tissue engineering, and drug delivery (Figure 5.18).

5.3.2.1 Proteins: Collagen

Collagen is the most abundant type of protein in the human body. The basic unit of collagen is a polypeptide consisting of the repeating sequence of glycine, proline, and hydroxyproline. This polypeptide combines with 12 others to form the left-handed triple helix structure in collagen. At least 22 different types of collagen have been identified so far in the human body. Collagen has been extensively investigated for various medical applications, including enzymatic degradability, unique physicochemical properties, mechanical properties, and biological properties. It can be processed into many different forms: sheets, tubes, sponges, powders, fleeces, injectable solutions, fibers, and dispersion. The use of collagen as a suture material dates back a millennium. One form of it, catgut, is still in use for surgery. Collagen is an attractive candidate for drug-delivery applications because of its biocompatibility, biodegradability, and its ability to be cross-linked by a variety of agents. Collagen shields and particles are used in ophthalmology to deliver drugs to the eyes. Collagen has also been used in grafts for corneal replacement, suture material, bandages, lenses, plugs, and viscous solutions for vitreous replacements during eye surgery. The high thrombogenicity of collagen makes it a potential candidate as a haemostatic agent. Currently it is used in haemostatic sealant for treatment of bleeding in cardiovascular and spinal surgical procedures (Sulzer-Spine Tech). Collagen sponges have been extensively investigated as wound and burn dressings. Collagen matrices can improve cellular adhesion and proliferation. Combined with proteoglycans, collagen is metabolically stable. It has been extensively investigated as an artificial skin, which accelerates wound healing. Because of its fibrous nature, collagen can withstand tensile loads. It has been investigated for applications that require structural integrity. Composites of collagen with hydroxyapatites have been investigated as scaffolds for bone tissue engineering. Despite the versatile properties of this natural polymer, only very few products based on collagen have gone clinical trials. The immunogenicity of collagen is a concern because it is dependent on the source and processing techniques. Other concerns include high cost of pure collagen, variability in the physicochemical properties, and degradation properties because of its source (animal) and processing technique. The threat of the disease transmission such as bovine spongiform encephalopathy is also concerning.

5.3.2.2 Proteins: Gelatin

Gelatin is essentially denatured collagen. It is prepared by the thermal denaturation of collagen, usually from animal skin and bones in the presence of dilute acid. Gelatin consists of

19 amino acids joined by peptide linkages. The enzymatic degradation of the gelatin results in the corresponding amino acids. The benefits of gelatin over collagen arise around the fact that gelatin does not show antigenicity and has high hemostatic properties. The harsh acidic or basic conditions used to make gelatin also eliminate many of the adverse properties associated with collagen, purifying the substance. Gelatin can be easily cross-linked by a variety of cross-linking agents. It forms a hydrogel capable of imbibing large quantities of water. The high cytocompatibility of gelatin also makes it a suitable candidate for tissue-engineering applications, particularly as delivery matrices for growth factors. Gelatin can be processed into membranes, micro spheres, or nanospheres. Gelatin has been extensively investigated in drug-delivery matrices. It has been shown to have ease of processability, biodegradability, and hydrogel properties of chemically cross-linked or polyelectrolyte complexes.

5.3.2.3 Proteins: Albumin

Albumin is the protein of highest concentration in blood plasma. The primary function of albumin is to carry hydrophobic fatty acid molecules around the bloodstream. Albumin consists of a single polypeptide chain and exists mainly as an α-helix. Albumin, like gelatin, can be easily processed into membranes, microspheres, or nanospheres because of its solubility and the presence of reactive functional groups along the polymer chain. Albumin has been investigated in coatings for biomaterials to improve their blood compatibility. It has also been investigated in matrices for intravascular drug-delivery systems, with the conclusion that it inhibits fibrinogen adsorption, platelet aggregation, and has high blood compatibility.

5.3.3 Other Natural Materials

Aside from pure proteins and polysaccharides there are other materials that have been utilized by researchers and medical device companies to replace tissues, reinforce healing tissues, or regenerate new tissues. These materials are presented in a variety of forms and have been used *in vitro* and *in vivo* with a great deal of success.

5.3.3.1 Calcium Phosphate

Calcium phosphate makes up a majority of the mineral present in bone and the calcified sections of cartilage, ligaments, and tendons. Hydroxyapatite, $Ca_{10}(PO_4)_6(OH)_2$, is the predominant calcium phosphate in these tissues.

Calcium phosphate is presented in many forms; these forms include amorphous calcium phosphate, tricalcium phosphate, brushite, octacalcium phosphate, and hydroxyapatite. These forms are listed in order of most soluble to least soluble. As solubility decreases, the mechanical strength of the calcium phosphate increases. This leaves tissue engineers with an important decision, to focus more on degradability or mechanics when it comes to scaffold fabrication.

5.3.3.2 Decellularized Tissue (Allografts and Xenografts)

One way to make sure that your scaffold is biocompatible and has the ability to influence cell behavior is to use actual tissue. Decellularized tissues, allografts and xenografts, are excellent scaffolds for tissue engineering. Allografts are tissues that come from cadavers and xenografts come from animal sources. They are biocompatible, biodegradable, and have the ability to affect cellular behavior (proliferation, differentiation, migration, etc.) through structural, biomechanical, and biochemical cues.[1–5] In addition these decellularized tissues are a template for the cells to produce tissue with a natural architecture.

After removal from the host, the tissue must first be decellularized. The presence of outside genetic material can lead to rejection and failure of the implant. Therefore, decellularization is extremely important for the success of the decellularized matrix, but the process does damage the extracellular matrix. The amount and type of damage depends on the decellularization technique used. The choice of decellularization technique depends on the density of the tissue, its level of cellularity, thickness and lipid content.[5]

Decellularization techniques can be divided into two main categories: chemical (including the use of enzymes) and physical. Chemical methods include the use of acids, bases, detergents, enzymes, and solvents.[3,5] Physical techniques include the use of force or pressure, freezing temperatures, and electroporation.[3,5]

Detergents work by sulublizing the lipid membranes of cells, unfortunately detergents can also be harmful to signaling proteins (which can help with differentiation of the seeded cells) and structural proteins such as growth factors (which are necessary for maintaining tissue mechanical properties). Sodium dodecyl sulfate (SDS) is a common detergent for dense tissues that has been used on a variety of tissues and organs including kidney, heart, vein, and the temporomandibular joint.[6–9] If it is used for too long a period of time or at too high a concentration, SDS can alter tissue mechanical properties and decrease growth factor and glycosaminoglycan content. The ionic nature of SDS makes it difficult to remove from the tissue without extensive washing. Triton X-100 is another detergent that is used in thick tissues such as heart valves.[10] Triton X-100 is not ionic, so it is not as harsh to proteins as SDS and therefore does a better job of preserving tissue structure and mechanical properties than SDS. Sodium deoxycholate (SD) is another ionic surfactant, like SDS, but it is milder to proteins than SDS. Unfortunately, its use can lead to the aggregation of DNA at the tissue surface; this can be alieviated by combining SD with a deoxyribonuclease I to break down the DNA.[11] 3-[(3-cholamidopropyl)dimethylammonio]-1-propanesulfonate (CHAPS) is zwitterionic (a dipole ion)m is not as harsh on protein as SDS, and is most effective on thinner tissues.[12]

Acids and bases have also been used for decellularization. Peracetic acid has been used on thin tissues. In some cases the mechanics of the tissues changed, the peracetic acid caused increases in modulus.[13] In other cases cell removal was not complete.[14] Basic calcium oxide alkaline solutions have been used with detergents to remove additional cellular material through reversible alkaline swelling, which is reversed with ammonium sulfate.[15] The swelling caused a decrease in glycosaminoglycan content and altered the viscoelastic properties.

Enzymes have been used with other decellularization techniques to increase their effectiveness. The enzyme trypsin is commonly used with ethylenediaminetetraacetic acid (EDTA) to break cell-matrix adhesions. Longer exposure increase its effectiveness but can also lead to damage to the matrix evidenced by decreases in elastin and collagen content.[16,17] DNases and RNases are effective nucleotide removal after cell lysis through by another technique, like use of detergents.[12,18] Collagenases can also be used for cell removal, but they can drastically decrease the mechanical integrity of the tissue. Collagenases are used in some cell isolation procedures to obtain primary cells for culture.

Acetone is used for lipid removal during decellularization, but it is a fixative that damages the tissue structure and forms crosslinks to increase mechanical properties.[7,19,20] Tributyl phosphate (TBP) is an organic solvent that has been used to decellularize dense tissues such as tendon.[21]

Increased hydrostatic pressure is one technique to remove cells through mechanical lysis of their membranes. Although it can effectively destroy cells, the DNA is still left behnd, requiring washing with a DNase.[22] The use of this treatment can lead to ice formation, which can damage the tissue structure.[23] This can be offset by increasing the temperature which can also cause tissue structure disruption.[23]

Freezing and then thawing the tissue is another technique used to lyse cells.[24,25] This technique causes only minor damage the tissue, so collagen and glycosaminoglycan contact and mechanical properties are similar to those before the treatment. Unfortunately, this process may leave behind a large amount of DNA material.[24] This may cause an immunogenic response *in vivo*.

Electroporation uses electric fields to open cell membranes, these disruptions can be temporary or permanent (leading to cell death) depending on the strength of the field and the amount of time the cell spends in the field. This technique can be applied to tissues for decellularization.[26] This technique uses probes to create the electric field (between the probes) so there are size limitations with this technique.[5]

5.4 METALS

Although they are not normally used in tissue engineering, metals are still a play a large role in biomedical engineering and are frequently placed in contact with damaged tissue as a structural support. Two of the most widely recognizable examples are the use of metallic stents within the cardiovascular system and the use of metallic implants in orthopedics. In both cases, the metal is in contact with living tissue and therefore must be biocompatible. The use of different coatings can also make them bioactive. In this section we will provide a brief introduction to metals, metallic structure, metal processing, and mechanics. For a more in-depth analysis of metals and their use in medical applications, please read *Biomaterials Science*, by Ratner et al., and *Materials Science and Engineering: An Introduction*, by Callister.[27,28] Both were consulted as sources for this chapter.

5.4.1 Metals: Bonding

Metals are materials that exhibit metallic bonding in the solid state. The free electron model of metallic bonding states that metal atoms are strong electron donors; they do not form ionic or covalent bonds. Instead, the atoms are arranged in a highly ordered, repeating, three-dimensional structure, and the valence electrons migrate around the atoms. This type of bonding creates a closely packed atomic crystal structure. Bond strength increases as the atomic cores and electron "gas" become tighter packed, which lowers the energy of the system (because the atomic cores are as close together as possible).

5.4.2 Metals: Structure

About 85% of all metals have one of three atomic packing structures: body-centered cubic (BCC), face-centered cubic (FCC), and hexagonal close-packed (HCP), a denser version of a simple hexagonal crystal structure. In FCC and HCP, every atom is surrounded by 12 nearest neighbors. This is the closest packing formation possible for spheres of uniform size. In these configurations, the atoms occupy 74% of the space. In BCC, every atom touches 8 neighbors (called an *eightfold coordination*). The atoms in this configuration occupy 68% of the space (Figure 5.19 and Table 5.1).

5.4.3 Metals: Crystals

When the periodic and repeated arrangement of atoms extends throughout the entirety of the specimen without interruption, the result is a crystal, where are unit cells interlock in the same way with the same orientation. Single crystals exist in nature, but they may also be produced artificially. However, they are difficult to grow and require a carefully controlled

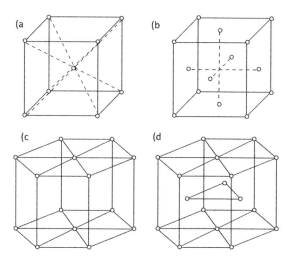

FIGURE 5.19 Metal crystal structures: (a) body-centered cubic (BCC), (b) face-centered cubic (FCC), (c) simple hexagonal, and (d) hexagonal close packed (HCP).

TABLE 5.1   Crystal Structures and Crystal Radii for Metals Commonly Used in Medical Implants

Metal	Crystal Structure	Uses
Chromium	BCC	Component of alloys for orthopedic implants
Iron	BCC	Component of steel for knee implants
Gold	FCC	Plating for stents, anti-cancer drugs, electronics
Nickel	FCC	Component of Nitinol in stents and alloys for orthopedic implants
Platinum	FCC	Electronic implants, stents, orthopedic implants
Magnesium	Simple Hexagonal	Component of alloys researched for orthopedic implants
Cobalt	HCP	Component of alloys for orthopedic implants
Titanium	HCP	Component of alloys for orthopedic and dental implants
Zirconium	HCP	Component in alloys used in joint replacements

BCC, body-centric cubic; FCC, face-centric cubic; HCP, hexagonal close packed.

environment. Most crystalline solids are polycrystalline, which means they are composed of many small crystals or grains. The small grains grow by the successive addition of atoms from the surrounding liquid to the structure of each crystal. Crystallographic orientation varies from grain to grain. There is atomic mismatch within the region where two grains meet and is called a *grain boundary.*

5.4.4 Metals: Imperfections

A dislocation within a metal is a linear or one-dimensional defect around which some of the atoms are misaligned. An edge dislocation occurs when the edge of an extra portion of a plane of atoms ends within the crystal. This is a linear defect. There is some localized lattice distortion around the dislocation line. Atoms above the dislocation line are squeezed together and those below are pulled apart (Figure 5.20).

A screw dislocation occurs when the upper front region of the crystal is shifted one atomic distance to the right relative to the bottom portion; the atomic distortion is a linear defect. The screw dislocation derives its name from the spiral or helical path or ramp that is traced around the dislocation line by the atomic planes of atoms.

Grain boundaries are interfacial defects. These boundaries separate two small grains, or crystals, that have different crystallographic orientations. Figure 5.21. There are different types of grain boundaries. The small-angle grain boundary occurs when the orientation mismatch is on the order of a few degrees. The tilt boundary is a small-angle grain boundary formed when the edge dislocations are aligned. The twist boundary is a small-angle grain boundary that is formed when arrays of screw dislocations are present.

5.4.5 Metals: Devices and Fabrication

Pins, screws, plates, replacements (hip, knee, vertebrae), and cages are among the metallic medical devices that are used mainly for orthopaedic applications. Metals are also used in oral and maxillofacial surgery for dental implants and craniofacial plates and screws.

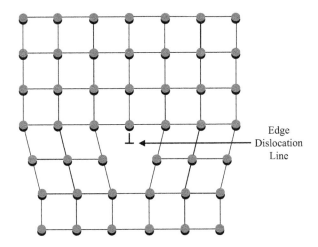

FIGURE 5.20   A two-dimensional schematic of an edge dislocation.

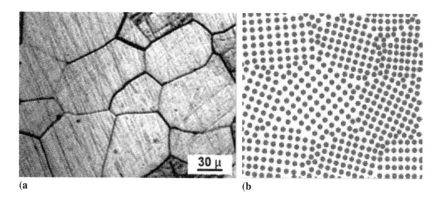

(a   (b

FIGURE 5.21   Micrograph showing grain boundaries and a diagram of different crystallites in a polycrystalline metal. (From Wikipedia, https://en.wikipedia.org/wiki/Grain_boundary.)

In cardiovascular surgery, metals are present in stents, artificial heart parts, pacemakers, balloon catheters, and valve replacements.

Implant manufacturers usually buy stock metal and form the implant to fabricate the device. The steps taken depend on the type of metal used because some alloys are difficult to machine. Basic fabrication methods for metal implants include investment casting, conventional and computer-based machining, forging, powder metallurgical processes, grinding, and polishing. Coatings have recently become popular because microporous and microporous coatings have been shows to alter cell behavior. They are also used to improve bonding after implantation. Alloy beads, fiber metal coatings, and sprays such as hydroxyapatite are among the types of coatings. Some of these techniques add "roughness" to the devices to improve cellular adhesion and elicit a cellular response, usually the growth of a new tissue. Porous coatings have been used to increase bonding with the metal implant and surroundings in press-fit hip implants, where the new bone can grow into the pores to increase bonding between the bone and implant. One problem that may arise is that motion and stress can cause the new bone to break while inside the pores, creating particles and loosening the implant.

5.4.6 Metals: Altering Properties

Steps are taken before device manufacturing to obtain metals with specific mechanical properties. Metallurgical and materials engineers use different hardening techniques, as well as different alloys, to obtain materials with the right strength for the application. The plastic deformation of a metal is caused by the motion of large numbers of dislocations. The easier it is for these dislocations to move, the less stress is required for the metal to deform; the harder it is for these dislocations to move, the more stress is required to plastically deform the metal. Therefore, reducing the mobility of dislocations enhances the mechanical strength. Restricting or hindering dislocation motion renders a material harder and stronger.

Strain hardening, or work hardening, is the process of making a ductile metal harder and stronger as it is plastically deformed. The temperature at which deformation takes place is "cold" relative to the absolute melting temperature of the metal. This is called *cold working*. It is sometimes convenient to express the degree of plastic deformation as the percentage of cold work (%*CW*). It is defined as:

$$\%CW = \frac{A_o - A_d}{A_o} \times 100$$

A_o is the original area of the cross section that experiences deformation, and A_d is the area after deformation. The dislocation density in a metal increases with deformation or cold work. The average distance of separation between dislocations decreases and dislocations are positioned closer together. On the average, dislocation-dislocation strain interactions are repulsive, so the motion of a dislocation is hindered by the presence of other dislocations. As the dislocation density increases, this resistance to dislocation motion increases. It is important to note that as a metal is cold worked, its hardness is increased but its ductility is decreased.

Annealing is a heat treatment in which a material is exposed to an elevated temperature for an extended time period and then slowly cooled. This is used to increase softness, ductility, and toughness, as well as to produce a specific microstructure. A variety of annealing heat treatments are possible. They are characterized by the changes that are induced. These changes are usually microstructural and are responsible for the alteration of the mechanical properties. Any annealing process consists of three stages. First, the material is heated to the desired temperature, then it is held or "soaked" at that temperature. Finally, it is cooled, usually to room temperature. Process annealing is a heat treatment that is used to negate the effects of cold work. It softens and increases the ductility of a previously strain-hardened metal. It is used during fabrication procedures that require extensive plastic deformation. This allows a continuation of deformation without fracture. Ordinarily a fine-grained microstructure is desired, and therefore the heat treatment is terminated before appreciable grain growth has occurred.

Alloying metals also alters their properties. Just like any other composite, alloys have a blend of the properties of their constituent components. Solid solution strengthening is a type of alloying that can be used to improve the strength of a pure metal. Atoms of one element are added to a crystalline lattice comprised of atoms of another. The alloying element will diffuse into the matrix, forming a "solid solution." The strength of a material is a measurement of how easily dislocations in its crystal lattice can be propagated. The dislocations create stress fields within the material. When solute atoms are introduced, local stress fields are formed that inhibit the motion of the stress fields caused by the dislocations. This increases in the yield stress of the material.

5.4.7 Metals: Types

There are several different types of alloys used in biomedical engineering. They include stainless steel, cobalt-based alloys, and titanium-based alloys.

5.4.7.1 Stainless Steel

Stainless Steel is labeled 316L (ASTM F138, 139). It is comprised of 60%–65% iron, 17%–19% chromium, and 12%–14% nickel, as well as minor amounts of nitrogen, manganese, molybdenum, phosphorous, silicon, and sulfur. The L stands for low carbon content. If the carbon content goes far beyond 0.03%, there is the risk of forming carbides. Carbides tend to precipitate at grain boundaries as $Cr_{23}C_6$, which depletes chromium content avavilable for chromium oxide formation and can possibly lead to corrosion.

Adding chromium leads to corrosion resistance and forms Cr_2O_3 (surface oxide). In its desirable form, 316L is FCC for both F138 and F139. There should be no BCC in the structure, and it should be free from sulfide stringers and other inclusions. Impurities could lead to pitting type corrosion at the metal-inclusion interface. The desirable metal is usually 30% cold worked and used in orthopaedic devices.

5.4.7.2 Cobalt-Based

Cobalt-based alloys include Haynes Stellite 21 (F75) and Haynes Stellite 25 (F90), which are Co-Cr-Mo alloys. ASTM F75's main attribute is corrosion resistance in chloride environments because of its bulk composition and the surface oxide (Cr_2O_3). This alloy has a long history in the aerospace and biomedical implant industries. F75 is cast into shape by investment casting. The alloy is melted at 1350°C–1450°C and then poured or driven into ceramic molds of the desired shape (e.g., femoral stems for artificial hips, oral implants, dental partial bridgework). Molds are made by making a wax pattern and then coating the pattern with a special ceramic. The wax is burned away and the ceramic mold remains, then molten metal is poured into the mold. Once the metal has solidified into the shape of the mold, the ceramic mold is cracked away and processing continues toward the final device. The other cobalt-based alloy, ASTM F90, is also known as Haynes Stellite 23 (HS-25), which is a Co-Cr-W-Ni alloy. Tungsten and nickel are added to improve machinability and fabrication properties. When annealed, its mechanical properties are similar to F75. When cold worked to 44%, the properties more than double.

5.4.7.3 Titanium-Based

The most common titanium-based alloys are implant biomaterials, specifically Cp titanium (ASTM F67) and extra-low interstitial (ELI) Ti-6Al-4V. The F67 CP Ti is 98.9%–99.6% titanium. Oxygen content of CP Ti affects its yield and fatigue strength significantly. At 0.18% oxygen (grade 1), the yield strength is about 170 MPa. At 0.40% (grade 4), the yield strength is about 485 MPa. ASTM F67 is used in dental implants. Typical microstructures are single-phase alpha (HCP) with mild (30%) cold work. Interstitial elements (O, C, N) in titanium and the 6AI-4V alloy strengthen the metal through interstitial solid solution strengthening mechanisms, with nitrogen having approximately twice the hardening effect of either carbon or oxygen.

The Ti-6Al-4V ELI alloy consists of Al, an alpha (HCP) phase stabilizer, and V, a beta (BCC) phase stabilizer. The 6Al-4V alloy used for implants is an alpha-beta alloy. There is increasing interest in the chemical land physical nature of the oxide on the surface of 6Al-4V, TiO_2. The oxide provides corrosion resistance and may also contribute to the biological performance of titanium at molecular and tissue levels, as suggested in the literature on osseointegrated oral and maxillofacial implants.

5.5 IMPORTANCE TO TISSUE ENGINEERING

The use of an appropriate material is critical for the fabrication of an implant that performs well both mechanically and biologically. There are a plethora of materials and fabrication methods available for these purposes. A tissue engineer has to know the mechanical and biological properties of the tissue that is being replaced and choose the material and structure that can most closely match them.

QUESTIONS

1. Describe the process of electrospinning. How can you change the diameter or orientation of the nanofibers produced by the process?

2. How can the surrounding environment alter the electrospinning process?

3. What is the glass transition temperature of a polymer, and why is it important?

4. What would happen if you implanted a polymer with a glass transition temperature higher than room temperature and lower than body temperature?

5. How does mixing or agitation speed effect microsphere or nanosphere size during fabrication?

6. How can you improve the strength of a metallic device?

7. Are chitin and cellulose readily degradable? If not what processing steps are necessary to make them degradable?

8. What is the difference between bulk erosion and surface degradation?

9. Why are polyphophazenes a unique type of synthetic polymer?

10. What does it mean when a polymer is crystalline?

REFERENCES

1. Vorotnikova E, McIntosh D et al. Extracellular matrix-derived products modulate endothelial and progenitor cell migration and proliferation in vitro and stimulate regenerative healing in vivo. *Matrix Biology.* 2010 29(8):690–700.
2. Bornstein P, Sage EH. Matricellular proteins: Extracellular modulators of cell function. *Current Opinion in Cell Biology.* 2002 14(5):608–616.
3. Gilpin A, Yang Y. Decellularization strategies for regenerative medicine: From processing techniques to applications. *BioMed Research International.* 2017 2017:9831534.

4. Allen RA, Seltz LM et al. Adrenal extracellular matrix scaffolds support adrenocortical cell proliferation and function in vitro. *Tissue Engineering, Parts A* 2010 16(11):3363–3374.
5. Crapo PM, Gilbert TW et al. An overview of tissue and whole organ decellularization processes. *Biomaterials.* 2011 32(12):3233–3243.
6. Nakayama KH, Batchelder CA et al. Decellularized rhesus monkey kidney as a three-dimensional scaffold for renal tissue engineering. *Tissue Engineering, Parts A.* 2010 16(7):2207–2216.
7. Lumpkins SB, Pierre N et al. A mechanical evaluation of three decellularization methods in the design of a xenogeneic scaffold for tissue engineering the temporomandibular joint disc. *Acta Biomaterialia.* 2008 4(4):808–816.
8. Guyette JP, Charest JM et al. Bioengineering human myocardium on native extracellular matrix. *Circulation Research.* 2016 118(1):56–72.
9. Schaner PJ, Martin ND et al. Decellularized vein as a potential scaffold for vascular tissue engineering. *Journal of Vascular Surgery.* 2004 40(1):146–153.
10. Meyer SR, Chiu B et al. Comparison of aortic valve allograft decellularization techniques in the rat. *Journal of Biomedical Materials Research Part A.* 2006 79(2):254–262.
11. Pellegata AF, Asnaghi MA et al. Detergent-enzymatic decellularization of swine blood vessels: Insight on mechanical properties for vascular tissue engineering. *BioMed Research International.* 2013 2013:918753.
12. Petersen TH, Calle EA et al. Tissue-engineered lungs for in vivo implantation. *Science.* 2010 329(5991):538–541.
13. Gilbert TW, Wognum S et al. Collagen fiber alignment and biaxial mechanical behavior of porcine urinary bladder derived extracellular matrix. *Biomaterials.* 2008 29(36):4775–4782.
14. Syed O, Walters NJ et al. Evaluation of decellularization protocols for production of tubular small intestine submucosa scaffolds for use in oesophageal tissue engineering. *Acta Biomaterialia.* 2014 10(12):5043–5054.
15. Mendoza-Novelo B, Avila EE et al. Decellularization of pericardial tissue and its impact on tensile viscoelasticity and glycosaminoglycan content. *Acta Biomaterialia.* 2011 7(3):1241–1248.
16. Schenke-Layland K, Vasilevski O et al. Impact of decellularization of xenogeneic tissue on extracellular matrix integrity for tissue engineering of heart valves. *Journal of Structural Biology.* 2003 143(3):201–208.
17. Rieder E, Kasimir MT et al. Decellularization protocols of porcine heart valves differ importantly in efficiency of cell removal and susceptibility of the matrix to recellularization with human vascular cells. *The Journal of Thoracic and Cardiovascular Surgery.* 2004 127(2):399–405.
18. Yang B, Zhang Y et al. Development of a porcine bladder acellular matrix with well-preserved extracellular bioactive factors for tissue engineering. *Tissue Engineering Part C: Methods.* 2010 16(5):1201–1211.
19. Jamur MC, Oliver C. Cell fixatives for immunostaining. *Methods in Molecular Biology.* 2010 588:55–61.
20. Cole MB, Jr. Alteration of cartilage matrix morphology with histological processing. *Journal of Microscopy.* 1984 133(Pt 2):129–140.
21. Cartmell JS, Dunn MG. Effect of chemical treatments on tendon cellularity and mechanical properties. *Journal of Biomedical Materials Research.* 2000 49(1):134–140.
22. Hashimoto Y, Funamoto S et al. Preparation and characterization of decellularized cornea using high-hydrostatic pressurization for corneal tissue engineering. *Biomaterials.* 2010 31(14):3941–3948.

23. Funamoto S, Nam K et al. The use of high-hydrostatic pressure treatment to decellularize blood vessels. *Biomaterials*. 2010 31(13):3590–3595.

24. Xing Q, Yates K et al. Decellularization of fibroblast cell sheets for natural extracellular matrix scaffold preparation. *Tissue Engineering Part C: Methods*. 2015 21(1):77–87.

25. Cortiella J, Niles J et al. Influence of acellular natural lung matrix on murine embryonic stem cell differentiation and tissue formation. *Tissue Engineering Part A*. 2010 16(8):2565–2680.

26. Phillips M, Maor E et al. Nonthermal irreversible electroporation for tissue decellularization. *Journal of Biomechanical Engineering*. 2010 132(9):091003.

27. Brunski JB. Classes of materials used in medicine: Metals. In: Ratner BD, Hoffman AS, Schoen FJ, Lemons JE (Eds.). *Biomaterials Science: An Introduction to Materials in Medicine*. San Diego, CA: Academic Press; 1996. pp. 37–50.

28. William D, Callister J. *Materials Science and Engineering: An Introduction*. New York: John Wiley & Sons; 1994.

CHAPTER 6

Fabrication

Various Techniques

6.1 INTRODUCTION

The success of a tissue-engineering project depends on a lot of different areas. The type of cells used, the use of growth factors, and the materials that the cells are seeded on and in the scaffold are all extremely important for the viability of the developing tissue. One area of equal importance is the structure of the scaffold used to house the cells. The architecture of the scaffold influences the chemical species that the cells are exposed to through the diffusion of materials through its pores. It can control the metabolic activity of the cells by subjecting cells to surfaces that are on par with the size of the seeded cells or much larger than the seeded cells. The architecture can limit or allow cell and tissue infiltration through pore size and pore interconnectivity. If a scaffold is too porous the mechanical strength may be compromised, leading to premature failure. In light of the importance of scaffold architecture a variety of techniques have been developed to produce a wide range of architectures to give cells different surfaces and pore sizes to ensure regenerative tissue success. In this section, we will discuss several techniques that create commonly used scaffolds in the area of tissue engineering.

6.2 ELECTROSPINNING

Electrospinning is a technique used to create polymeric fibers with diameters in the nanometer range. This process involves the ejection of a charged polymer fluid onto an oppositely charged surface. One of the first investigations into the flow of conducting liquid through a charged tube with a counterelectrode some distance away was conducted by Zeleny.[1] His work introduced a precursor to electrospinning called *electrospraying*. In these experiments, an electrical charge was added to low viscosity, aqueous electrolyte solutions with high electrical conductivity. Adding an electrical charge to these solutions caused them to spray toward to the counterelectrode. As they traveled through the air, the droplets evaporated in the air.

Electrospinning is just like electrospraying, except the solution is of a much higher viscosity because of the presence of the polymer in the solution. In electrospinning, the charge is applied to a polymer solution or melt and ejected toward a grounded or oppositely charged target. In electrospinning and its precursor, electrospraying, the surface tension and viscoelastic forces of the polymer solution are at odds with the electrical field around the solution coming out of the syringe.[2] The viscoelastic forces and surface tension want to keep the polymer solution as a droplet at the tip of the syringe. The electric field wants to pull the droplet toward the oppositely charged or grounded target (as seen in electrospraying). If the strength of the electric field is slightly larger than the viscosity and surface tension the polymer solution gets drawn from the droplet, deforming it into a "Taylor cone" at the tip of the syringe (Figure 6.1) and a narrow, charged jet is ejected from the tip of the Taylor cone. The jet whips through the air evaporating the solvent (or cooling the polymer if a polymer melt is used) on its way to the grounded or oppositely charged substrate. When it reaches the substrate, the solvent is gone and all that is left is a nonwoven mat of fibers. One of the first electrospun substances was cellulose acetate. A patent for the process was given to Formhals in 1934.[3]

The concentration of the solution, viscosity of the solution, and the entanglement of the polymer chains cause a fiber to be extruded from the Taylor cone. They maintain the cohesiveness of the solution and are important for electrospinning because without it you have electrospraying. The polymer jet starts off as a straight line but becomes unstable because of the repulsive forces from charges in the polymer jet. This causes electrically driven bending instabilities within the jet, forcing it to move around in a spiral and stretch.[4] The stretching aids in solvent evaporation and greatly decreases the fiber diameter. Together, all of these actions create nanoscale thin fibers, which land randomly onto the grounded or oppositely charges target (Figure 6.2).

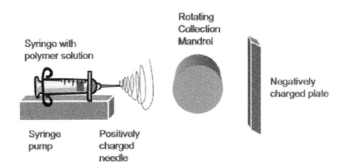

FIGURE 6.1 Schematic for electrospinning. (From McKeon-Fischer, K., *Creation and Characterization of Several Polymer/Conductive Element Composite Scaffolds for Skeletal Muscle Tissue Engineering*, Virginia Polytechnic Institute and State University, Blacksburg, VA, 2012.)

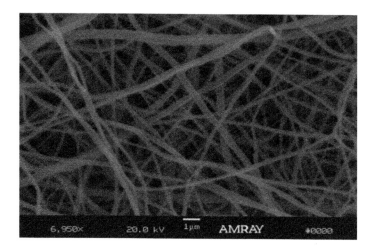

FIGURE 6.2   Electrospun gelatin nanofibers.

This process creates fibers with extremely small diameters in the submicron range. The fiber diameter can be altered by changing the distance between the syringe (your polymer source and the grounded or oppositely charged target), the polymer concentration, and the voltage. The arrangement of the nanofibers onto the target can be adjusted by employing various external mechanical or electrostatic forces. The mechanical properties of the fiber mat can be altered by changing the diameter and orientation of the fibers.

All of the parameters that affect the electrospinning process can be split into different groups: polymer solution properties (parameters that directly affect the polymer source), processing parameters (parameters that effect the fabrication of the nanofibers), and environmental parameters (parameters that effect the area in which you are electrospinning).[1,3,4–7] Electrospinning parameters in the area of polymer solution properties include solution viscosity, polymer molecular weight, polymer concentration, surface tension, solution conductivity, and the dielectric effect of the solvent. Increasing the polymer concentration of the electrospinning solution increases the viscosity and leads to a larger number of polymer chain entanglements in the solution. Both of these lead to greater resistance of the polymer jet to stretching, creating higher diameter fibers. This allows the bending instability to set in much later in the travel path toward the target, which means the spread of the jet is lower and has a smaller deposition area onto the target. If the polymer concentration is lowered, this lowers the viscosity and shifts control of the process from viscosity and entanglements to surface tension due to less polymer chain entanglement, where beads on the fiber will form.

Increasing the conductivity of the solution increases the charge transfer by the electrospinning jet. It also allows for the formation of bead-free fibers under conditions that usually cause beads. Higher conductivity also creates a higher deposition area of the nanofiber matrix and lower fiber diameter, as well as higher bending instability because of the increased jet path. It also lowers the critical voltage required for electrospinning. Conductivity can be increased by increasing the ion content of the solution which increases the stretching of the fibers. Higher dielectric constant solvent reduces bead formation, increases the bending instability, increases the deposition area, and decreases the fiber diameter. A lower dielectric constant solvent may interfere with the polymer solubility and might lead to the formation of beads.

Electrospinning-processing parameters that affect nanofiber fabrication include voltage, distance from needle to collector, flow rate, needle/orifice diameter, and type of collector. Increased voltage increases the stretching force that is applied to the fibers, allowing better orientation and alignment molecules. It may also accelerate the fibers reducing the time of flight of the jet to collector, which might provide less time for the polymer molecules in the jet to orient. Increased voltage can increase the crystallinity of the resultant fiber if the flight time for the jet is sufficient. A decrease in distance will lead to increased electrical potential, which may lead to an acceleration of the polymer jet but provides shorter path length. There may not be sufficient time for the solvent to evaporate, resulting in intra- and interlayer-bonded fibers. An increase in collector distance will lower the diameter. Increasing the distance beyond the optimum value the electrostatic field strength yields a higher diameter of the collected fibers and poor quantity of fiber collection and eventually the process ceases.

Increasing flow rate increases the fiber diameter or form beads there is more polymer than the applied potential can handle. It will also prevent complete solvent evaporation. Decreasing the flow rate will starve the Taylor cone, which may cause it to recede inside the needle or orifice, causing fiber defects. Lower amounts of fiber will be collected. A smaller needle/orifice diameter will lead to less clogging during the electrospinning process, partially because of less exposure of the solution to the atmosphere. Extremely small inner diameter makes the polymer solution extrusion difficult, and droplet size decreases as well. The surface tension of the droplet increases and the critical voltage of the electrospinning process to start is increased.

Electrospinning environmental parameters include humidity, pressure, and type of atmosphere. Humidity affects solvent evaporation; at higher humidity, water might condense on the fiber while being electrospun, which results in altered morphology. At extremely low humidity, evaporation rate may increase, which could lead to the clogging of the needle. Decreased pressure will result in rapid bubbling of the solvent at the tip, higher discharge from the needle tip, leading to an unstable jet initiation, and little to no resistance of the electrospinning atmosphere, thus direct discharge occurs.

6.2.1 Special Types of Electrospinning

Electrospun nanofibers can have a wide range of morphologies based on the technique used. As stated previously, the nanofibrous mats produced by electrospinning can have nanofibers that are oriented in one direction or randomly arranged. Groups have added nanoparticles such as nanohydroxyapatite powder, gold nanoparticles, or carbon nanotubes to polymer solutions to imbed them into the nanofibers. If the diameters of the particles are large enough, they can protrude from the nanofibers. Another technique used to create unique nanofibers is coaxial electrospinning. In this technique one nanofiber is produced inside of another nanofiber, each nanofiber has an inner core with a sheath surrounding it (Figure 6.3).[8] Coaxial electrospinning allows you to produce nanofibers

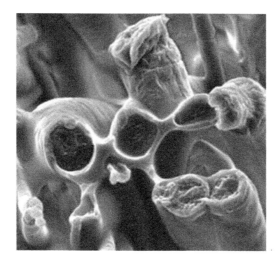

FIGURE 6.3 Scanning electron micrograph of coaxial electrospun nanofibers. (From McKeon-Fischer, K.D. et al., *J. Biomed. Mater. Res. A.*, 99, 493–499, 2011.)

composed of two materials with different solubilities in organic or aqueous solvents.[9] This creates nanofibers with unique properties or controlled release of a chemical factor (the chemical must pass through two layers instead of one).

6.2.2 Applications of Nanofibers in Tissue Engineering

Electrospun nanofibers have been used in many different structures. Researchers have altered their fabrication process to form larger structures from the nanofibers, electrospun nanofibers on top of larger structures or combine nanofibrous mats to form larger structures. Nanofibers have been electrospun into tubular structures.[10–13] This is typically done by electrospinning onto a rotating drum. The orientation of the nanofibers that make up the tube is controlled by the speed of the drum. Increasing the rotational speed aligns the nanofiber perpendicular to the tube long axis. These scaffolds have been investigated for use as artificial blood vessels and in bone scaffolds.[12,14]

Another larger structure created by nanofibers is the nanofiber thread. These threads can be used in woven scaffolds for fibrous tissues such as tendon, ligament, and muscle. In one technique, the polymer is electrospun into a liquid; the nanofibers are then dragged through the liquid, the shear forces created by moving the nanofibers through the liquid lead to nanofiber alignment.[15] A variation of this theme electrospins into a water-filled dish with a drain at the bottom.[16] The water and nanofibers are drawn down the drain and the sheer force of water on the nanofibers aligns them. The aligned nanofiber thread is then collected below the drain. In another technique, nanofibers are electrospun between the tips of two oppositely charged metal blades; this technique forms a bundle or yarn of nanofibers.[17]

Other groups have formed similar structures but called them *yarns*. One process for nanofibrous yarns has been developed by Ko et al.[18] The steps in this process include alignment by blowing air along the nanofibers, drawing of the material over a rotating mandrel (to increase alignment) drawing through a set of spinning drums, and fiber twisting. Other groups have formed similar structures by electrospinning onto needle tips and manually transferring the bundled fibers onto a rotating collecting drum or electrospinning onto two rings and spinning the rings to twist and bundle the fibers.[19,20]

Other groups have combined multiple nanofibrous mats to form larger three-dimensional structures. Freeman et al. developed a technique that involves nanofiber sintering.[21,22] In this technique, the researchers combined multiple nanofibrous mats by stacking them or winding one mat around into a cylinder and then heating the nanofibers to the polymer glass transition temperature. This allows the nanofibers to polymers in each layer to bind with polymer in a neighboring layer without melting the polymer and losing the nanofibrous structure.

6.3 MICROSPHERES/NANOSPHERES

Nanospheres are polymeric spheres that are hundreds of nanometers in diameter; microspheres are tens to hundreds of microns in diameter (Figure 6.4).[23] Their tiny size and ability to absorb or bind to drugs or growth factors (through surface chemistry) make them ideal vehicles for drug or growth factor delivery. They also create pores of comparable size when they are bound together by sintering. Because of their spherical shape, this process creates interconnected pores throughout the structure. The spheres can be poured into any mold and sintered to create porous scaffolds of any shape.

Polymeric micro/nanospheres can be created by emulsion solvent diffusion. To do this, a polymer is dissolved into a volatile organic solvent, such as chloroform, ethyl acetate, or methylene chloride. This solution is then poured into an aqueous phase with a surfactant or stabilizer and agitated. The agitation forces the polymer phase into small droplets within the aqueous phase. As the speed of agitation increases the size of the droplet decreases; typically stirrers are used to make microspheres, while nanospheres are made with a sonicator. The nanospheres are then collected by evaporating the solvent

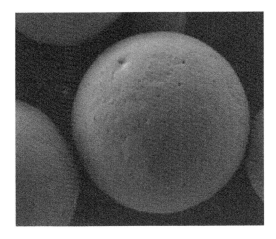

FIGURE 6.4   Scanning electron micrograph of polymeric microsphere with hydroxyapatite. (From Lv, Q., et al., *J. Biomed. Mater. Res. A* 91, 679–691, 2009.)

or dilution with water. Sphere size (and density) is also controlled by the amount of polymer added to the surfactant or stabilizer solution. In the past these structures have been used in drug delivery or tissue engineering.[24–29]

Drugs and growth factors may be added to the organic or aqueous phase to incorporate them into the nanospheres. To improve mechanical properties, nanoparticles of materials, such as calcium phosphate (usually in the form of hydroxyapatite), are added. Calcium phosphate can also enhance osteodifferentiation and osteoblast proliferation within tissue engineered bone scaffolds.[30] Changing the sphere size can also alter the strength of the scaffold, level of porosity, and pore size distribution. The density of microspheres can be altered by creating hollow spheres, referred to as lighter-than-water (LTW) microspheres.[23] LTW microspheres are created by bubbling the polymer solution and then pouring it into the stabilizer (or surfactant). The microspheres formed around the bubbles of air become hollow and float to the top. The others fall below the liquid surface (as normal). By combining these LTW microspheres with normal solid (also called heavier-than-water or HTW) microspheres you can control the buoyancy of your constructs, which is useful in rotating cell culture.

6.4 HYDROGELS

Hydrogels are three-dimensional swollen networked structures that can provide shock absorption and viscoelastic properties and are investigated for cartilage replacement. They are networks of joined polymer chains, which are soft and malleable, and swell when introduced to water, which increases viscoelasticity (Figure 6.5). These materials are able to swell and retain the volume of the adsorbed aqueous medium in their three-dimensional swollen network when placed in a compatible aqueous medium. They can revert back to a collapsed state when the water is removed and reversibly swell again in the presence of water (Figure 6.5). Materials for hydrogel formation include natural materials (plant, animal origins such as collagen/gelatin and proteoglycans, and chemically modified) and synthetic polymeric materials. Hydrogels generally swell to an equilibrium value of 10%–98% at physiologic temperature, pH, and ionic strength. A dried hydrogel imbibing at least 20 times its own weight of the aqueous media while retaining its original shape could be referred to as *superabsorbent*. In some cases, it can be as much as 1000 times the weight of the polymer. Hydrogels may respond uniquely to changes in external environmental conditions such as ionic strength, electromagnetic radiation, pH, and temperature. The type of salt used for the preparation of buffer, solvent used as the medium, photoelectric stimulus, and external stress

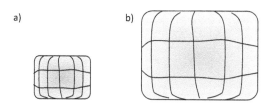

FIGURE 6.5 Hydrogel in a collapsed state (a) and a swollen state (b).

also influence hydrogel behavior. Hydrogels exhibit both liquid-like and solid-like properties. The liquid-like properties result from the fact that the major constituent (>80%) is water, whereas the solid-like properties are attributed to the network formed by the crosslinking reaction. Hydrogels behave like elastic solids. There is a remembered reference configuration to which the hydrogel returns after being deformed for a long time. Synthetic polymeric hydrogels are generally three-dimensional swollen networks of hydrophilic homopolymers or copolymers covalently or ionically crosslinked. The original polymeric hydrogel network was developed by Wichterle and Lim in Czechoslovakia in 1954. It consisted of a copolymer of 2-hydroxyethyl methacrylate (HEMA) and ethylene dimethacrylate (EDMA), and was used as contact lenses. It was not until the 1960s when the versatility of synthetic polymeric hydrogels was visualized from a commercial point of view.

The classification of hydrogels depends on their physical structure and chemical composition. There are neutral hydrogels, ionic hydrogels, and swollen interpenetrating polymer networks (IPNs). Polymeric hydrogels are classified in accordance to their monomeric composition based on the method of preparation (homopolymeric hydrogels and copolymeric hydrogels). The chemical constituent of monomers used in the preparation also plays an important role in classifying the hydrogel (neutral, anionic, cationic, ampholytic). It is all based on the presence of ionic charges on the monomer. Hydrogels are also classed as amorphous or semi-crystalline materials based on their physical nature.

Homopolymers are polymer networks derived from a single species of the monomer, which is the basic structural unit comprising of any polymer. Homopolymers can have crosslinked or uncross-linked skeletal structure, which depends on the nature of the monomer and polymerization technique. Hydrogels are used in slow drug-delivery devices and contact lenses. Cross-linked homopolymeric hydrogels of poly(hydroxyalkyl methacrylates) PHEMA are among the most widely studied and used of all synthetic hydrogel materials. Uncross-linked homopolymers include poly(ethylene glycol) (PEG) and poly(vinyl alcohol) (PVA). PEG and PVA have been widely used in biomedicine and agricultural applications.

Copolymeric hydrogels are composed of two or more different monomer species (Figure 6.6). They have at least one hydrophilic component, arranged in a random, block,

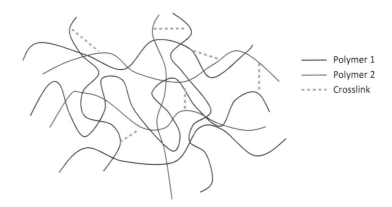

FIGURE 6.6 A drawing of the molecules in a copolymeric hydrogel.

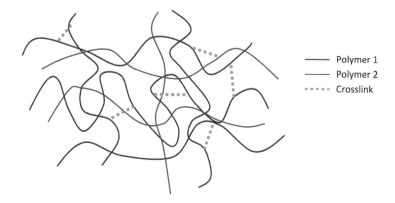

FIGURE 6.7   A drawing of the molecules in n interpenetrating network. Polymer 1 is crosslinked and surrounding polymer 2.

or alternating configuration along the chain of the polymer network. The number and arrangement of hydrophobic components can alter properties such as degradation rate.

Interpenetrating polymer networks (IPN) have two independent synthetic or natural polymer components contained in a network (Figure 6.7). One of the components is a crosslinked polymer, and the other is a non-crosslinked polymer.

Neutral hydrogels (non-ionic hydrogels) have no charged groups. They can be homopolymeric or copolymeric networks and swell to equilibrium when the osmotic pressure of the solvent is balanced with the subchain stretching energy. They collapse and swelling of neutral hydrogel networks occur normally as a result of change in the environmental temperature.

Ionic hydrogels (polyelectrolytes) are prepared from monomer's accompanying ionic charges, which can be positive (cationic), negative (anionic), or a combination of both (ampholytic). The inclusion of charged species in the polymer backbone enhances the stimuli responsive properties, used in actuator applications. Anionic hydrogels are either homopolymers of negatively charged acidic or anionic monomers or copolymers of an anionic monomer and a neutral monomer. Anionic hydrogels are known to exhibit a marked increase in the swelling ratio with increase in the environmental pH. Cationic hydrogels are either homopolymers of positively charged basic monomers or copolymers of cationic and neutral monomers. Polyampholytic hydrogels are macromolecules capable of possessing both positively and negatively charged parts in the polymer network. The net charges on these materials can be changed to achieve the desired functional property by changing the monomeric composition of the feed mixture. This is used in biomedical applications including sustained drug-delivery systems.

During formation, hydrogels are usually crosslinked chemically or physically. In chemically crosslinked hydrogels, polymer chains are connected by covalent bonds, while polymer chains of physical gels are connected through non-covalent bonds, such as van der Waals interactions, ionic interactions, hydrogen bonding, or hydrophobic interactions.

The extent of cross-linking in the hydrogel network is referred to as cross-linking density. Increased cross-linking density will increase the resistive force to chain elongation, which reduces the degree of equilibrium swelling and makes the hydrogel more brittle.

6.5 3D PRINTING

One scaffold fabrication technique that has gained popularity within the last decade is three-dimensional (3D) printing. 3D printing is actually a catch-all phrase that encompasses several types of additive manufacturing. Additive manufacturing describes "technologies that build 3D objects by adding layer-upon-layer of material."[31] The most common materials are polymers, typically thermoplastice, but other materials can be used in additive manufacturing including metal, wood, concrete, ceramics, and natural materials like cross-linkable proteins or polysaccharides.

There are currently 11 types of 3D printing available today. They are fused deposition modeling (FDM), stereolithography (SLA), direct light processing (DLP), selective laser sintering (SLS), direct metal laser sintering (DMLS), selective laser melting (SLM), electron beam melting (EBM), material jetting (MJ), drop on demand (DOD), laminated object manufacturing (LOM), and binder jetting.[32,33]

6.5.1 Fused Deposition Modeling (FDM)

Fused deposition modeling (FDM) is one of the most commonly used 3D printing techniques. This technique was first developed by Scott Crump when he realized that he could build 3D objects automatically using a hot glue gun and a robotic XYZ gantry system.[34] This led to the creation of Stratasys, a global leader in 3D printing technologies. FDM machines create objects from thermoplastics (in either filament or molten form). The polymer is heated and extruded through a nozzle along a pattern determined by a computer file. The object is built layer by layer, from the bottom to the top. Objects with hollowed out or overhanging regions may need to have removable support structures printed to prevent the collapse of the object.

Before the object is built by FDM the object is designed using 3D CAD software. The CAD model is then divided into slices or layers. These layers are read by the printer which then builds each layer of the object. This type of printing typically has the lowest amount of resolution, limited by the nozzle size. FDM typically uses thermoplastics but can also print ceramics, metals, and wood if they are combined with a binder material. Because of their relatively low price, researchers have modified FDM machines to print hydrogels by extruding the polymer solution, instead of a molten polymer, and then cross-linking it layer by layer with UV light.

6.5.2 Stereolithography

Stereolithography (SLA) is a modern form of a classic printing technique. Lithography is actually a very old way to make prints repeatably; it has been around for over 200 years. Lithography was a printing method invented in Germany by Alois Senefelder in 1798.[35] The technique is based on the immiscibility of oil and water. Designs formed with an oil-based medium (such as crayon) on limestone. The limestone is then wetted, the water is absorbed everywhere except the areas covered by the crayon. A roller is then used to apply an oily ink to the stone. The ink only adheres only to the drawing and not the wet stone. A piece of paper is then pressed against the design and the print is made.

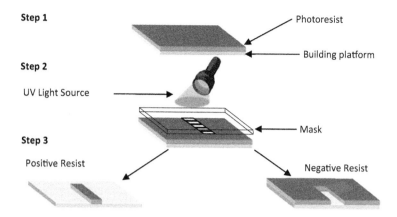

FIGURE 6.8 Basic steps in photolithography using positive and negative photoresists. (Based Freeman, J.W. et al., Nanofabrication techniques, In: Gosalves, K.E., Haberstadt, C.R., Laurencin, C.T., Nair, L.S. (Eds.), *Biomedical Nanostructures*, John Wiley & Sons, Hoboken, NJ, pp. 3–24, 2008.)

Later this technique was used to create 3D images using masks, light, and resins which would then cross-link into solids when exposed to light. Optical lithography was developed when Rick Dill developed a set of mathematical equations to describe lithography in the "Dill papers" during the 1970s.[36] The first lithography modeling program SAMPLE was developed in 1979 by Andy Neureuther.[36] The technique is still the same as the original lithography, use a mask to force the medium to develop in certain areas and make it difficult for it to develop in others. Photolithography transfers designs onto the surface of a photoresist material[36,37] (Figure 6.8). The process has been refined and miniaturized and is used to form semiconductors and biosensors. To date photolithography has become one of the most successful technologies in the field of microfabrication. Briefly a light is shined on a photoresist material. To make precise shapes a mask is placed over the material so that only certain areas are exposed to the light and allowed to crosslink. Once the cross-linking is finished the uncross-linked material is rinsed away leaving behind your device. If this is submerged into the photo resist again, you can build larger objects. By changing the mask layer by layer, you can create more complex designs. Different versions of this process include contact printing, where the mask touches the photoresist surface and proximity printing, where the mask is microns away from the surface. Some processes use a positive photoresist solution where exposure to the light makes the resist more soluble and allows it to wash away leaving behind the area covered by the mask. There have been different variations of lithography throughout the years. We will describe several of them in the following sections.

6.5.2.1 Limitations of Photolithography

Current photolithography techniques use a projection-printing system where the image of the mask is reduced in size and projected onto a thin film of the photoresist material.[36,37] The resolution that the system is based on optical diffraction limits set in the Rayleigh equation.[37]

$$R = \frac{k_1 \lambda}{NA}$$

where k_1 is a photoresist constant, λ is the wavelength of the light source, and NA is the numerical aperture of the lens. In this technique the smallest available feature size is approximately equal to the wavelength of the light used, λ (theoretically the lower limit is $\lambda/2$). So to decrease the size of a structure to micro- or nanoscaled shorter wavelength light must be used, which can be more expensive and difficult.

SLA uses the same basic principles as photolithography. The technique shines light onto a photoresist material to cross-link it and produce structures layer by layer, from the bottom up. The main difference is that instead of using a mask SLA uses a precision laser that is guided by the layers produced from the sliced CAD file. Because the printer controls where the laser will go there is no need for a mask. After each layer is formed by exposure to the laser, the object is dropped into the bath of photoresin by one layer to allow another layer to be formed on top of the previous one. Most SLA machines use a solid state UV laser. The path of the laser light is controlled using mirrors called *galvanometers*, or *galvos*. One galvo is positioned on the *x*-axis, and another galvo is on the *y*-axis. They move to aim the laser beam across the photoresin to form each layer of the device.

When the printing finished the object needs to be rinsed with a solvent and exposed to UV light for further curing. Only certain polymer solutions can be used in this process (not all are biocompatible). A number of researchers develop their own biocompatible photoresins. The use of laser light to form the layers makes SLA rapid and very precise; SLA has better resolution than FDM.

6.5.3 Direct Light Processing

Direct light processing (DLP) is very similar to SLA. Both use photo cross-linking to make objects layer by layer. The difference is that instead of UV laser light (as in SLA), DLP uses more traditional sources such as light-emitting diodes (LEDs) or arc lamps. Each layer is formed at one time using one flash of light using a digital screen that projects the image of that layer. The projection is shined onto the polymer using an array of mirrors called a digital micromirror device (DMD). The ability to expose the polymer resin to the entire layer at once makes DLP faster than SLA. The use of screen means that the projections are composed of pixels, giving DLP lower resolution than SLA. The use of standard light sources instead of lasers means that this technique is ammendable to the use of hydrogels of both synthetic and natural materials without burning them. Printing the entire layer at once eliminates creep of extruded polymer solution after it is extruded, but before it is cross-linked.

6.5.4 Selective Laser Sintering

In selective laser sintering (SLS), a high power CO_2 laser is used to fuse, or sinter, particles together to form a solid structure. This techniques is also called *Powder Bed Fusion*. and it works for powdered polymers, metals, glass, and ceramics. In SLS, a blade or wiper deposits a very thin layer of the powedered material onto the platform. Afterward, the CO_2 laser runs across the surface of the platform in a pattern determined by the CAD file; as in SLA the laser is positioned by a set of galvos. This sinters selected particles into a solid piece. When the sintering of that layer is complete, the platform drops by one level, the blade deposits another layer of powder onto the object and the process is repeated. The unsintered powder acts as a support material for the build.

As in SLA, the use of the laser gives this technique better resolution than FDM. This technique also places a layer of unprocessed material on top of a sintered layer to form the next layer, as seen in SLA. In fact, the only real difference between the two techniques is that SLA uses a powder, whereas SLA uses a liquid resin.

6.5.5 Direct Metal Laser Sintering

Direct metal laser sintering (DMLS) is very similar to SLS. It uses a laser to heat metal powders to the point of fusion (without melting). After the fabrication of a layer a wiper adds another layer of powder over the build for the heating of the next layer. Although this technique is similar to SLS, DMLS requires the use of support structures during printing to prevent warping of the object. This technique can be used with alloys such as stainless steel and cobalt chrome. As you can imagine because of the use of metal DMLS has limited applications in tissue engineering.

6.5.6 Selective Laser Melting

Selective laser melting (SLM) is just like SLS, a powder is laid down by a wiper or blade. A laser heats the powder in a specific pattern, guided by a sliced CAD model. After the layer is finished, the building platform drops, an new layer of powder is laid down and the process is repeated. The difference between SLM and SLA is that except instead of sintering the powder, as in SLS, SLM melts the powder, this typically leads to the production of stronger objects than those produced by SLS. SLM also takes place under inert or noble gas.

6.5.7 Electron Beam Melting

Electron beam melting (EBM) is another technique that is similar to SLM. However whereas SLM uses a laser, EBM uses an electron beam. In addition, SLM can be performed in standard atmosphere and pressure under a gas, but EBM must be performed in a vacuum. EBM can only be performed on poders of conductive materials, such as metals.

6.5.8 Material Jetting (MJ)

Material jetting (MJ) has aspects of FDM and SLA. Like SLA the materials used are photo cross-linked to form a solid, like FDM the material for one layer is deposited on top of the previous layer. The process works like an inkjet printer. A layer of the "ink" is printed out and cross-linked with UV light, according to the sliced CAD model. The platform is then lowered and the process repeated. This technique was initially used by some of the early labs that performed bioprinting. Researchers took inkjet printers and added a z-axis component to get them to drop between printed layers so that 3D printouts could be produced. The inks could include cells and instead of printing different colors the machines would print different cell types, materials, or both. Because of its similarity to inkjet technology, objects are produced point by point, not in drawn out filaments like FDM.

6.5.9 Drop on Demand

Drop on demand (DOD) uses two inkjets to lay down waxy materials. One material forms the object, typically a mold, and the other lays down a support material thet can be dissolved or melted away after fabrication.

6.5.10 Laminated Object Manufacturing

Laminated object manufacturing (LOM) fuses (or laminates) large pieces of polymer or paper together, layer by layer, until the final object is formed. This is unique from other 3D printing techniques because it builds objects from preformed layers of material. A sheet is transferred to the platform and then cut to the desired shape by a laser or blade. After cutting the platform drops, and another layer is placed on top, cut, and then bonded to the layer below using heat and pressure. This process is repeated until the object is formed. This process is rapid, but it is not capable of high resolution and can be used with sands, polymers, metals, and ceramics.

6.5.11 Binder Jetting

Binder jetting (BJ) uses powdered material to print objects, like SLS and SLM. Unlike these techniques, BJ uses a bonding agent to hold the particles together instead of sintering or melting them together. A powder layer is followed by a layer of liquid bonding agent. For each layer the building platform is lowered, as in SLS and SLM. This is repeated in BJ.

6.6 IMPORTANCE TO TISSUE ENGINEERING

Human tissues and organs are extremely complex. Their architectures contain different fiber sizes and fiber arrangements. Different tissues contain different structures and potentially different materials giving them each different mechanical and biological properties. Technological advancements allow us to reproduce different aspects of tissue architecture with a variety of different techniques. Using nanofibers, or hydrogels or nanospheres, we can design scaffolds with architectures or mechanical properties similar to what the cells experience *in vivo*. With 3D printing, researchers can produce scaffolds for specific defects. As technologies advance we are closer to producing implants that can more closely mimic real tissue for seamless replacement and regeneration.

QUESTIONS

1. Describe the differences between scaffolds produced by electrospinning and scaffolds produced by FDM 3D printing.

2. How can one produce nanospheres instead of microspheres or lighter than water microspheres instead of heavier than water microspheres?

3. What is the difference between a copolymer hydrogel and an interpenetrating network?

4. Name the different ways molecules can bind together to produce hydrogels.

5. Name and describe five different 3D printing techniques.

6. Want is the importance of the Rayleigh equation in photolithography?

7. What is coaxial electrospinning?

8. How does humidity affect the electrospinning process?

9. Electrospinning and stereolithography are based off of what original techniques?

10. Hydrogels are designed to absorb large amounts of what?

REFERENCES

1. Zeleny J. Electric discharge from points. *Physical Review.* 1917 9:562–563.
2. McKeon-Fischer K. *Creation and Characterization of Several Polymer/Conductive Element Composite Scaffolds for Skeletal Muscle Tissue Engineering.* Blacksburg, VA: Virginia Polytechnic Institute and State University. 2012.
3. Formhals A, inventor; Apparatus for producing artificial filaments from material such as cellulose acetate. United States patent law. United States of America patent 1975 504. 1934.
4. Reneker DH, Yarin AL et al. Bending instability of electrically charged liquid jets of polymer solutions in electrospinning. *Journal of Applied Physics.* 2000 87:4531–4547.
5. Freeman JW, Laurencin CT et al. Nanofabrication techniques. In: Gosalves KE, Haberstadt CR, Laurencin CT, Nair LS (Eds.). *Biomedical Nanostructures.* Hoboken, NJ: John Wiley & Sons; 2008. pp. 3–24.
6. Huang ZM, Zhang YZ et al. A review on polymer nanofibers by electrospinning and their applications in nanocomposites. *Composites Science and Technology.* 2003 63:2223–2253.
7. Yarin AL, Koombhongse S et al. Taylor cone and jetting from liquid droplets in electrospinning of nanofibers. *Journal of Applied Physics.* 2001 90(9):4836–4846.
8. McKeon-Fischer KD, Flagg DH et al. Coaxial electrospun poly(ε-caprolactone), multiwalled carbon nanotubes, and polyacrylic acid/polyvinyl alcohol scaffold for skeletal muscle tissue engineering. *Journal of Biomedical Materials Research: Part A.* 2011 99(3):493–499.
9. Saraf A, Lozier G et al. Fabrication of nonwoven coaxial fiber meshes by electrospinning. *Tissue Engineering Part C Methods.* 2009 15(3):333–44.
10. Panseri S, Cunha C et al. Electrospun micro- and nanofiber tubes for functional nervous regeneration in sciatic nerve transections. *BMC Biotechnology.* 2008 8:39.
11. Wang W, Itoh S et al. Influences of mechanical properties and permeability on chitosan nano/microfiber mesh tubes as a scaffold for nerve regeneration. *Journal of Biomedical Materials Research.* 2008 84(2):557–66.
12. Lee SJ, Liu J et al. Development of a composite vascular scaffolding system that withstands physiological vascular conditions. *Biomaterials.* 2008 29(19):2891–2898.
13. Teo WE, Kotaki M et al. Porous tubular structures with controlled fibre orientation using a modified electrospinning method. *Nanotechnology.* 2005 16:918–924.
14. Andric T, Freeman JW (Eds.). *Fabrication of Mineralized Osteon-like Scaffolds.* Pittsburgh, PA: BMES Annual Meeting; 2009.
15. Smit E, Buttner U et al. Continuous yarns from electrospun fibers. *Polymer.* 2005 46:2419–2423.
16. Teo W, Gopal R et al. A dynamic liquid support system for continuous electrospun yarn fabrication. *Polymer.* 2007 48:3400–3405.
17. Teo WE, Ramakrishna S. Electrospun fibre bundle made of aligned nanofibres over two fixed points. *Nanotechnology.* 2005 16:1878–1884.

18. Ko F, Gogotsi Y et al. Electrospinning of continuous carbon nanotube-filled nanofiber yarns. *Advanced Materials*. 2003 15(14):1161–1165.

19. Wang X, Zhang K et al. Enhanced Mechanical performance of self-bundled electrospun fiber yarns via post-Treatments. *Macromolecular Rapid Communications*. 2008 29(10):826–831.

20. Dalton PD, Klee D et al. Electrospinning with dual collection rings. *Polymer*. 2005 46:611–614.

21. Wright LD, Young RT et al. Fabrication and mechanical characterization of 3D electrospun scaffolds for tissue engineering. *Biomedical Materials*. 2010 5(5):055006.

22. Andric T, Wright L et al. Fabrication and characterization of three-dimensional electrospun scaffolds for bone tissue engineering. *Journal of Biomedical Materials Research Part A*. 2012 100A(8):2097–2105.

23. Lv Q, Nair L et al. Fabrication, characterization, and in vitro evaluation of poly(lactic acid glycolic acid)/nano-hydroxyapatite composite microsphere-based scaffolds for bone tissue engineering in rotating bioreactors. *Journal of Biomedical Materials Research Part A*. 2009 91(3):679–691.

24. Borden M, Attawia M et al. Tissue-engineered bone formation in vivo using a novel sintered polymeric microsphere matrix. *The Journal of Bone and Joint Surgery*. 2004 86(8):1200–1208.

25. Borden M, Attawia M et al. Tissue engineered microsphere-based matrices for bone repair: Design and evaluation. *Biomaterials*. 2002 23(2):551–559.

26. Borden M, El-Amin SF et al. Structural and human cellular assessment of a novel microsphere-based tissue engineered scaffold for bone repair. *Biomaterials*. 2003 24(4):597–609.

27. Khan Y, Yaszemski MJ et al. Tissue engineering of bone: Material and matrix considerations. *Journal of Bone and Joint Surgery*. 2008 90(Suppl 1):36–42.

28. Khan YM, Katti DS et al. Novel polymer-synthesized ceramic composite-based system for bone repair: An in vitro evaluation. *Journal of Biomedical Materials Research Part A*. 2004 15 69(4):728–737.

29. Laurencin CT, Ambrosio AM et al. Tissue engineering: Orthopedic applications. *Annual Review of Biomedical Engineering*. 1999 1:19–46.

30. Kim K, Fisher JP. Nanoparticle technology in bone tissue engineering. *Journal of Drug Targeting*. 2007 15(4):241–252.

31. AM A. AM Basics: Amazing AM, LLC; 2013. Available from: http://additivemanufacturing. com/basics/.

32. Insider D. The 9 different types of 3D printers: 3D insider; 2018. Available from: http://3dinsider. com/3d-printer-types/.

33. Yusef B. 3D Printing Technology Guide: 10 Types of 3D Printing Technology-Simply Explained: All3DP; 2018. Available from: https://all3dp.com/1/types-of-3d-printers-3d-printing-technology/.

34. Moutch M. FDM 3D printing inventor Scott Crump enters Minnesota inventors hall of fame: 3D printing industry; 2014. Available from: https://3dprintingindustry.com/news/ fdm-3d-printing-inventor-scott-crump-enters-minnesota-inventors-hall-fame-26876/.

35. Henshaw M. First impressions: The early history of lithography-A comparative survey. *Artonview*. 2003 33(33–38).

36. Mack CA. Optical lithography modeling. In: Sheats JR SB (Eds.). *Microlithography Science and Technology*. New York: Marcel Dekker; 2006. pp. 109–170.

37. Ronse K. Lithographie optique—une vue historique. *Comptes Rendus Physique*. 2006 7(8):844–857.

CHAPTER 7

Cellular Biology in Tissue Engineering

7.1 INTRODUCTION

In the past few decades, there has been an exponential burst of research activity dedicated to the fields of tissue engineering and regenerative medicine. Transplantation therapy and clinical trials have been major contributors and hallmarks of these two fields. Unfortunately, the number of organs available for transplants has been experiencing a gradual decrease year after year. This is where tissue engineering comes into play. The entire purpose of this science is to generate organs from stem cells, which can then ultimately be transplanted back into the patient. This would fix the problem of organ shortage and help people obtain the proper treatment in time. However, the use of stem cells constantly faces political and ethical challenges, which is why researchers rely on new inventions and techniques by which they can obtain and harvest these incredible cells.

In this chapter, the reader will be introduced to some basic tissue biology and how these tissues collaborate with other components of the body. Next, we will start to inspect some of the choices associated with tissue engineering. This section will explain the various types of cells that can be used and the sources from which they are derived from. The next two sections will introduce primary cells and cell lines and their similarities and differences. Both primary cells and cell lines possess important distinctions, and it is pivotal to understand what types of cells are appropriate for a given research study. The section on cell rejection will give a brief background on immunity and explain some of the complications associated with transplants if they get rejected. Following the section on cell rejection, the reader will learn about the uses of stem cells and tissue engineering and some of the various techniques that are currently available. Finally, the stimulatory influences section is comprised of four different parts. First, we will give a brief overview of the various types of stimulations and then we will go into more detail in each of the respective sections. In the growth factors, mechanical, thermal, and electrical stimuli sections we will explain the role of these stimulations and their use in the clinic. In the end, the reader should have a general idea of how vast this field is and understand the various technologies that are available.

7.2 BIOLOGY AND BACKGROUND

7.2.1 Introduction

The term *regenerative medicine* is a term that is often closely related with tissue engineering. The objective of this system is to merge the fields of life sciences with engineering to stimulate body regeneration by controlling the internal biological environment. One of the main reasons why regenerative medicine has become so recognized is because it provides alternatives to organ transplantation. Organs are limited resources and immune responses against transplants often evoke the immune system to respond negatively to foreign materials. The emerging field of regenerative medicine works to correct these two important predicaments in addition to many others. It relies on the use of an abundant source of stem cells, biomaterial scaffolds, and growth factors to achieve these goals.

7.2.2 What Are Stem Cells?

Stem cells are natural pools of cells found in our body that work continuously to replenish the specialized cells that are required for our normal functioning of our bodies. Most stem cells are present in our bone marrows, which differentiate endlessly to produce the required amount of new blood cells in our bodies. Other stem cells present in our bodies differentiate to generate specialized cells to replenish used or damaged cells.

Stem cells have the capacity to differentiate into various cell types throughout the body during the early growth of humans or animals. Along with this, in many tissues these stem cells act as a sort of internal repair system by differentiating without any limit to help restore other cells for the entire duration of human or animal life cycle. When a stem cell divides into a new cell, it has the capacity to either remain as a stem cell or become a more specialized cell such as a heart cell or a lung cell or a brain cell.

Stem cells can be distinguished from other cells as they exhibit two special traits. Firstly, they are uncommitted cells and are capable of self-renewal. This is one of the fundamental properties of a stem cell. Secondly, they can differentiate into various specific cell lineages under appropriate stimuli. For instance, in some organs such as the bone marrow, the stem cells continuously differentiate and replenish damaged and worn out cells whereas in organs such as the heart, they only differentiate under unique conditions.

Stem cells can be categorized broadly into three different types: totipotent cells, pluripotent cells and multipotent cells. Totipotent cells are by far the most important and most versatile of stem cells. In human and animal development, they are derived from early embryos and each cell possesses the capacity to grow into a new organism. Totipotent cells have the potential to give raise to virtually all types of human cells. These cells are produced during the early stages of embryonic development and within a few days, totipotent cells can divide and create multiple duplicates of the same totipotent cell.

During embryonic development, the totipotent cells can give raise to the second type of stem cells known as the *pluripotent cells*. Pluripotent stem cells are often termed as "true" cells. These cells however, do not have the capacity to produce an entire organism but can further differentiate into much more specialized cells such as a nerve cell or a red blood cell.

One type of pluripotent stem cells is known as *embryonic stem cells* (ESCs). ESCs are known as immortal cells and have an unlimited developmental potential. These cells can differentiate into various types of cells required by the human body. ESCs exhibit limitless capabilities in research that spans over from basic research to transplantation therapies for diseases ranging from heart disease to Parkinson's to leukemia and help in providing better treatment outcomes for these diseases.

ESCs are derived from embryos that are in the developmental stage before the implantation stage in the uterus. Five days after the embryo's development, the very first differentiation of the cells occurs. This allows the formation of blastocyst that contains two layers of cells, an outer and an inner layer. The outer layer is called the *trophectoderm* and is committed to form the placenta upon implantation. The inner layer of cells is called the inner cell mass (ICM). This layer of cells possesses the ability to produce any cell type present in the body. After the implantation of the embryo in the uterus, these cells then lose their limitless developmental abilities.

However, if the ICM is harvested from the blastocyst prior to the implantation stage, and cultured in appropriate laboratory conditions, these cells can continue to proliferate endlessly and retain their potential to differentiate into any cell in the body. The second type of pluripotent stem cells were identified when the ICM undergoes further cell division and forms two layers; the lower layer, which is called the *hypoblast*, will form the yolk sac and the upper layer of the ICM tissue will form the epiblast.[1] Epiblast stem cells (EpiSCs) are pluripotent stem cells that give raise to cells present in all of the three embryonic germ layers as follows:

- **Ectoderm:** This germ layer gives raise to brain, spinal cord, nerves, hair, skin, teeth, sensory cells of the eyes, nose, mouth and pigment cells.

- **Mesoderm:** This germ layer gives raise to muscles, blood, blood vessels, connective tissues, and the heart.

- **Endoderm:** This germ layer gives raise to the gut (pancreas, stomach, liver, and other associated organs of the gut), lungs, bladder, eggs, and sperm.

Next type of pluripotent stem cells is known as embryonic germ (EG) cells. These cells are derived from the gonads of postimplantation fetuses. EG cells possess similar characteristics to EpiSCs cells. They are also capable of forming the three germ layers (ectoderm, mesoderm, and endoderm) required for development of various cells in our bodies. Limited research and data are available for EG cells as the isolation of these cells are questionable. Significant research is required to further understand the complete potential of these cells and to prevent unwanted outcomes such as tumors or abnormal development.

The third type of pluripotent stem cells are known as embryonic carcinoma (EC) cells. These are "stem cells" that occur in unusual germ cell tumors called *teratocarcinomas*. They are also known as malignant counterparts of ESCs. These cells found in teratocarcinomas and are differentiated stem cells that occur in tumors. EC cells have been used extensively in research to investigate how stem cells identify different pathways of differentiation during embryonic development. Upon using of EC cells, various technologies were designed to derive totipotent ES cells from mouse blastocyst. This in turn led to the isolation of human ES cells from their respective blastocysts.

Recent advances in the last few decades of research in stem cells has led to the identification of few more types of stem cells, namely induced pluripotent stem cells (iPSCs), somatic cell nuclear transfer stem cells (SCNTs), and region-selective epiblast stem cells (rsEpiSCs). These types of stem cells are further discussed next.

- **Induced Pluripotent Stem cells (iPSCs):** These cells are obtained from "genetic reprogramming" of adult stem cells to obtain pluripotent patient-specific cell lines. These cells are genetically manipulated to express genes and factors, which allow the cells to maintain the properties of ESCs. iPSCs have provided researchers with a promising tool to derive disease specific stem cells to study and design possible treatments for degenerative disorders.

- **Somatic Cell Nuclear Transfer Stem Cells (SCNT):** These cells are derived from inserting a somatic (body) cell nucleus into an enucleated egg (an egg in which the nucleus is removed). This is then forced to divide to form an embryo. The embryo continues to grow normally until the stem cells from it can be harvested. SCNTs have the properties of ESCs; however, they are more like iPSCs. SCNT stem cells have successfully been produced in mice and nonprimate animals, such as monkeys, successfully. However, with human's cells successful development of SCNTs have proved to be challenging and only so far been reported with fetal or infant somatic cells.[2]

- **Region-selective epiblast pluripotent stem cells:** As indicated previously, we know that ESCs are isolated from ICM in the blastocyst stage of the embryo. These cells possess the ability to virtually differentiate virtually into any cell type. Because of this ability, ESCs have provided valuable insights in the field of developmental biology and regenerative medicine. Further insights led to the identification of another type of stem cells known as EpiSCs. These cells set themselves apart from ESCs as they possess unique molecular, cellular, and functional characteristics. Extensive research by Wu et al., has led to the identification of a new type of EpiSCs. By incorporating appropriate culture medium and inhibition of WNT signaling led to high colonies of pluripotent stem cells with reduced tumorigenic potential. These cells when implanted in postimplantation embryos *in vitro* resulted in grafting, mainly in the posterior parts of the epiblast. The grafted cells are known as region-selective pluripotent stem cells (rsEpiSCs). These cells will potentially allow the study of early events in human development.[3] rsEpiSCs are known to possess high clonogenicity and low tumorigenic properties when compared to ESCs and EpiSCs.

Once the embryonic stage of development is completed, these cells lose their unrestricted ability to develop into all cell types present in the body. These cells then lose their pluripotency and can only grow into certain types of cells in the body. Lastly, the third type of stem cells is known as multipotent stem cells. Multipotent cells can also develop into more than one cell type. However, these cells have two limitations

- their ability to differentiate, and
- their limited numbers in the body.

Examples of multipotent cells are those cells that are present in the brain. They can convert into different neural cells and glia or hematopoietic cells, which in turn can give raise to several cell types. However, these cells do not possess the ability to create brain cells. Similarly, bone marrow also contains multipotent cells that have limited potential to generate into all blood cell types. Thus, multipotent cells are considered as adult stem cells because their limited ability to produce one or more cell lines. Unlike pluripotent cells, these cells are more limited in their capacity to differentiate and give rise to specialized cells.

Multipotent stem cells are of two types, mesenchymal cells (MSCs) and hematopoietic cells. Mesenchymal stem cells generate specialized cells that belong to our skeletal tissues such as adipocytes (fat cells), chondrocytes (cartilage), and osteocyte (bone cells). MSCs are originally found in bone marrow, cord blood, placenta, and adipose tissues. Human MSCs isolated from bone marrow have been shown to differentiate into a variety of cell types both *in vivo* and *in vitro*. However, the bone marrow contains limited amounts of MSCs.

Hematopoietic stem cells were one of the very first stem cells to be identified. They are adult cells that are most commonly populated in bone marrow. These cells function by generating all other blood cell types in the body including myeloid and lymphoid lineages of blood cells.

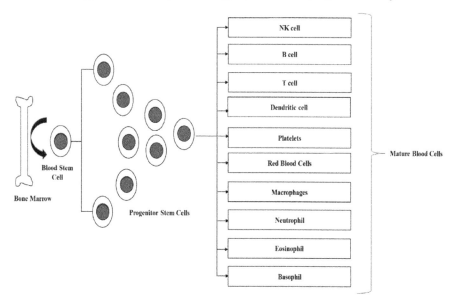

The figure shows all the blood cell types that are generated from a hemopoietin stem cells in the bone marrow (Table 7.1).

TABLE 7.1 Types of Stem Cells

Stem Cell	Where Do they Come From?	What Cells Can They Form?	Advantages	Limitations and Disadvantages
Totipotent Stem Cells	These cells are derived from a zygote cell when an oocyte is fertilized by the sperm.	These cells have the potential to give raise to virtually all human cells in the body.	Because these cells possess the ability to differentiate into any human cell, they display an enormous therapeutic value. These cells are the ideal candidates for various cell and gene therapies and as well as in the field of transplantation.	Totipotent cells remain in the state of totipotency for a short period of 4 days. After the zygote divides into an 8-stage cell state or higher, these totipotent cells begin to lose their potency. Hence, the biggest and formidable challenge that researchers encounter is the ethical concerns that revolve around the harvesting techniques of these totipotent fetal cells.
Pluripotent Stem Cells	ESC – These cells have unlimited development potential. These cells are derived from the inner cell mass (ICM) of a blastocyst. EpiSCs – These cells are harvested when the ICM undergoes further cell division. The ICM forms two layers and EpiSCs are harvested from the lower layer which forms the "epiblast." EG cells – These stem cells are derived from gonads of postimplantation fetuses. These cells possess similar characteristics to EpiSCs and can differentiate into cells of all the three germ layers. EC cells – These cells are "stem cells" that are isolated from unusual germ cell tumors teratocarcinomas. iPSCs – These cells are obtained from genetic reprogramming of adult cells to generate patient-specific cell lines. They are modified so that these cells can express properties of pluripotent stem cells. SCNT – These stem cells are reprogrammed from the blastocyst that was formed by using a somatic (body) cell and an enucleated egg (nucleus is removed). rsEpiSCs – These cells derived from the subpopulation of cells present in the posterior part of the postimplantation epiblast. These cells when injected into embryos *in vitro* led to grafting in the posterior parts of the epiblast. These grafted cells were found to be region-selective pluripotent stem cells.	These cells can differentiate into cells from various cell lines in our body. EpiSCs can form cells in all the three germ layers – ectoderm, mesoderm, and endoderm. EG cells have similar characteristics to EpiSC cells. They are also capable of differentiating into all cells of the three germ layers (ectoderm, mesoderm and endoderm). Because iPSCs are derived from adult tissues and do not require the use of embryos to harvest these cells. They can be designed to suit patient-specific needs.	ES cells can be grown in large quantities in laboratories and can be manipulated to differentiate into various cells. EC cells have been extensively used in research to identify how stem cells distinguish different pathways of differentiation during embryonic development. iPSCs are cells that have been genetically forced to express certain genes so that they can maintain the properties of a pluripotent stem cell. Researchers indicate that SCNT stem cells have potential use in regenerative medicine. rsEpiSCs and their discovery has led researchers to speculate about the profound impact it will have on the study of pluripotent stem cells, mammalian development, and regenerative medicine.	As these cells are not patient specific, there is a high chance that they may be rejected in immune suppressed patients if used for transplantation. Harvesting of embryonic stem cells again raise ethical concerns as these cells are derived from human embryos. Current research in iPSCs uses viral vehicles to bring about this forced change (genetic reprogramming) in the cells. This can sometimes cause cancers.

(Continued)

TABLE 7.1 (*Continued*)   Types of Stem Cells

Stem Cell	Where Do they Come From?	What Cells Can They Form?	Advantages	Limitations and Disadvantages
Multipotent Stem Cells	Mesenchymal cells – These cells differentiate into several cell types such as bone, muscle, cartilage, and other similar tissues. Hematopoietic cells – These cells are most commonly found in the bone marrow and can differentiate into all types of blood cells in the body.	These cells are found as undifferentiated cells in our bodies.	These cells can differentiate into only a few cell lines. Therefore, they are much easier to control because they have limited self-renewal capacity. The use of multipotent cells in research is less controversial. If these cells are used to generate required cells and tissue for transplantation, there is no chance of immune rejection if matched to the correct donor as these stem cells are derived from the same donor.	They are found in very small numbers in the body and are very difficult to find except for stem cells found in cord blood and in bone marrow. The most important limitation of multipotent stem cells is that they are able to differentiate into only those types of cells from the body part that they were found from. Multipotent stem cells are usually very difficult to grow in large quantities outside the body.

Abbreviations: EC, embryonic carcinoma cells; EG, embryonic germ cell; ESC, embryonic stem cell; iPSCs, induced pluripotent stem cells; SCNT, somatic cell nuclear transfer stem cell.

Stem cells or progenitor cells have expressed potential use in various aspects of the medical field. Research and investigations are under way for the use of stem cells as potential choice of treatment option.

Extensive research with stem cells has been conducted, which has led to positive results in various areas of regenerative medicine. However, these cells and their cultures are yet to be incorporated as standard of care. This is because stem cells are still in their preclinical stages and have so far only shown limited success in various animal models. As of now, the implementation of these results and their therapeutic prognosis in humans are still in their nascent stages.

Few other challenges that stem cells and their researchers encounter are as follows.

- Harvesting stem cells are not always ethically safe. Many ethical constraints surround the collection and culturing process that are involved when using stem cells on a large scale.

- Stem cells are collected mostly by invasive methods, which might lead to complications when received from the donor.

- Wide-scale application, production of stem cells, and laws to regulate the use of stem cells in research are still developing along with the research currently being conducted.

Stem cell transplantation has been used to study regenerative diseases of stroma, bone, adipose tissues, tendon and ligaments, cartilage, and cardiac muscle. Figure 7.1 illustrates some of therapeutic uses of stem cells and various applications of cell transplantation. These cells can further be used as potential drugs and as a part of gene therapies to treat a wide variety of diseases.

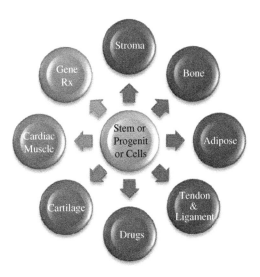

FIGURE 7.1   Cell transplantation.

7.3 CHOICE OF CELLS FOR USE IN TISSUE ENGINEERING

Before we begin any discussion on tissue engineering using human cells we must pay some attention to the choice of cells for *in vivo* use. When dealing with tissue engineering, there are many cells that are qualified experimental candidates. Some of the more recognized cells include the ESCs, which possess the ability to differentiate into potentially any lineage. There are also adipose-derived stem cells, bone mesenchymal stem cells, placental, and umbilical cord cells. Each of these cells functions in a unique way and serves in an integral purpose in regenerative medicine.

7.3.1 Bone Marrow–Derived Mesenchymal Stem Cells

One of the most recognized types of stem cells is the bone marrow–derived mesenchymal stem cell (BM-MSC). Mesenchymal stem cells (MSCs) are self-renewing and multipotent cells capable of differentiating into multiple cells including osteocytes, chondrocytes, adipocytes, hepatocytes and myocytes, neurons, and cardiomyocytes. MSCs reside in the stromal compartment of bone marrow and play an important role in providing stromal support for hematopoietic stem cells. This was identified with the help of pioneering studies conducted by Friedenstein et al.[4] MSCs comprise of only 0.001%–0.01% of total population of nucleated cells present in the bone marrow.[5] Initially MSCs were discovered in bone marrow, but recent research indicates the presence of MSCs in fat, epidermis, and cord blood.

One of the drawbacks of MSCs is that they lack tissue specific characteristics, but with the right influence signals they can differentiate into specialized cells. MSCs can be easily isolated, and with the right laboratory conditions, they can be expanded to very large numbers. These cells can be cultured in such a way that they do not lose their differentiation capacities for many generations. MSCs have generated great interest in the field of tissue engineering and regenerative medicines. Various pre-clinical and clinical trials with MSCs are in progress to identify and test the therapeutic value of MSCs in various degenerative diseases.

For instance, when treating patients for bone and cartilage disease, adult BM-MSCs are generally the best treatment choice because these cells have demonstrated that they are able to differentiate from a basic marrow cell population to an entire osteogenic lineage and thus have been used to catalyze repair of bone defects.[6–8] These mesenchymal stem cells can be isolated from the bone marrow colony-forming unit–fibroblastic (CFU-F)[4] and then be differentiated to other osteogenic lineages.[5,9]

Bone marrow cells are a very complex mixture of cells and thus require a more defined starting cell population to be isolated from the mixture.[10,11] Ultimately, these cells can be extracted from the marrow and used to enhance materials like the filler that is used for stabilizing artificial joints or for joining large defects in bone that would normally be impossible to heal naturally.[12]

7.3.2 Cord-Derived Stem Cells

As the name suggests, these cells are obtained from the embryo umbilical cord (UC) of humans. The UC contains two UC arteries (UCAs) and one UC vein (UCV). Both the arteries and veins are embedded within a specific mucous connective tissue known as Wharton's Jelly (WJ) and is covered by the amniotic epithelium.

One of the most pioneering discoveries was the identification of fibroblast-like cells from the WJ of the umbilical cord by McElreavey et al.[13] These UC cells were reported to have a similar surface phenotype and multipotency properties of MSCs.

UC is considered as medical waste and hence the collection of UC-MSCs is noninvasive. These MSCs are harvested by a painless procedure as compared to other methods of harvesting MSCs from humans.[14] They are also reported to have faster self-renewal properties in comparison with other MSCs. UC-MSCs have the ability to differentiate into the three germ layers (ectoderm, mesoderm, and endoderm), thereby possessing the capacity to differentiate into any one of these cell lineages.[14] These stem cells have been reported to accumulate in damage tissues or inflamed regions and promote repair and modulate tissue time response.[14]

Much research and focus has been shifted to umbilical cells since the discovery that cord-derived cells contained MSCs. Analysis of the gene expression of cord cells has revealed that cord cells have similarities to bone marrow stem cells.[15] Both cells are able to differentiate into adipocytes, osteoblasts,[16] hepatocytes, and neuronal-like cells.[17]

The potential for cord cells to act like bone marrow cells would serve as a great therapeutic advantage in treatment. This would provide a much larger pool and availability of stem cells. Moreover, the use of UC-MSCs could be used as an alternate source of MSCs because the differentiating function of bone marrow–derived stem cells decreased with age.[18,19] Finally, it is important to note that unlike ESCs, cord cells have the least ethical constraints and exhibit immunomodulatory properties. This is mainly because they are clinical by-products and involves no invasive methods to obtain them.[16,17]

7.3.3 Amniotic Membrane–Derived Stem Cells

Amniotic membrane is one of the components of the placenta. This membrane is present to protect the fetus during pregnancy and helps provide additional nutrients to the fetus. Amniotic membrane is comprised of three layers: a single epithelial layer, a thick basement membrane, and an avascular mesenchyme. Amniotic fluid present within the amniotic membrane contains a large heterogeneous cell population.

Two types of cells can be derived from the amniotic membrane and amniotic fluid, amniotic membrane stem cells (AMSCs) and amniotic fluid stem cells (AFSCs). AFSCs show great promise for future clinical applications. These are an ideal source of cells that provide easy access either during or after the pregnancy, requires simple isolation, and amplification of stem cells.

These cells can differentiate into various cell types, has immunomodulatory effects, and lack major ethical concerns. AFSCs can be used in transplantation techniques and can provide new treatment options for patients who have had ischemic strokes. However, much investigation is required to understand the complete potential of AFSCs and AMSCs.

7.3.4 Placenta-Derived Stem Cells

Further research in stem cells led to the identification of a new type of stem cells. These stem cells have limitless potential as determined by researchers in the field of regenerative medicine. Various types of stem cells such as embryonic, fetal, and adult stem cells exhibit different method of self-renewal programs.[20] These self-renewal programs change over time. Other ventures of research indicated that the ESCs with high telomerase activity were identified in the amniotic fluid.[21] However, the stem cells found in the amniotic fluid are of small quantities and cannot be used for transplantation.

Placenta is a rich and consistent source of fetal mesenchymal stem cells.[22–28] Placenta plays an important role in regulating the feto-maternal tolerance. Therefore, at birth preservation of placenta is important as because the only opportunity at which we can preserve these fetal autologous stem cells. Placenta mesenchymal stem cells (P-MSCs) are found to exhibit profiles that are like those found in ESCs.

One of the most important aspects of regenerative medicine is to identify an ethically safe source of stem cells. As discussed previously, we know that other stem cells present ethical issues with their use in research. Placenta-derived mesenchymal stem cells however do not pose this ethical constraint as placental is considered as medical waste and is available in large quantities.

P-MSCs can differentiate into the three germ layers (ectoderm, mesoderm, and endoderm) and thereby possess the ability to differentiate into various types of cells in our bodies. Presently, cord-derived MSCs are used in transplantation therapies with bone marrow–derived cells. Current findings suggest that placenta-derived stem cells can be of greater use than C-MSCs to provide aid in immunological conditions.

Various preclinical studies have been conducted in different areas of medicine such as liver, heart, pulmonary, bone diseases, and neurological diseases. They have also been used to explore the field of tissue engineering.

Human P-MSCs have found to exhibit neuroprotective properties after stroke in rats. When rats were treated with P-MSCs, vascular endothelial growth factor (VEGF), hepatocyte growth factor (HGF), and brain-derived neurotrophic factor (BDNF) levels in ischemic brain were found to have been elevated, as compared to the rats who served as controls in this study.[24] P-MSCs when transplanted into a mice model with Alzheimer's disease had higher levels of β-amyloid degrading enzymes, reduced levels of proinflammatory cytokines and increased levels of anti-inflammatory cytokines when compared to phosphate-buffered saline controls, slower progression of Alzheimer's pathology, and improved memory function.[25]

Placenta-derived mesenchymal stem cells have been investigated as cell therapies in liver diseases. P-MSCs have been revealed have shown the greatest potential for hepatogenic differentiation and proliferation *in vitro*. P-MSCs that were derived from the chorionic plate (the segment of the chorionic wall which attaches to the uterine lining) have found to express higher levels of hepatocyte growth factor differentiation.[26]

Extensive investigations with P-MSCs in pancreatic disease has led researchers to find that they possess the capacity to develop into insulin-producing cells.[27] They also have the ability to produce islet-like cell clusters, which led to the restoration of normoglycemia cycles when transplanted into streptozotocin-induced diabetic Balb/C mice.[28]

P-MSCs have also found to be useful in heart disease. A fragment of the human amniotic membrane was utilized onto the left ventricle of rats that have undergone ischemia through left anterior descending coronary artery ligation. Results of this study indicated that the amniotic membrane onto ischemic rat heats significantly reduced postischemic cardiac dysfunction once the rats presented higher values of left ventricle ejection fraction, fractional shortening, and wall thickening when echocardiographic examinations were performed.[29]

In the medical area concerning pulmonary diseases, a single center, nonrandomized, dose-escalation phase Ib trial was conducted with human patients who presented with moderately to severe idiopathic pulmonary fibrosis. The patients enrolled in this study received P-MSCs via peripheral vein and were followed for 6 months. The study demonstrated that the values measured after 6 months of follow-up revealed that all parameters measured during the study (forced vital capacity and diffusing capacity for carbon monoxide; 6-minute walk distance, gas exchange assessed by PaO_2, and lung fibrosis score as assessed by high resolution computed tomography chest) showed no evidence of worsening fibrosis. No side effects were reported in patients who received P-MSCs injection in this study.[30]

Fetal (early) chorionic stem cells as a treatment method was studied in a murine osteogenesis imperfecta (brittle bone disease) model. This study used intraperitoneal injections of P-MSCs in neonates exhibiting osteogenesis imperfecta, which revealed a decrease in fractures, increased bone ductility and bone value, and upregulated endogenous genes that are involved in endochondral and intramembranous ossification.[31] In the field of tissue engineering, P-MSCs are being investigated using various biomaterials, all which revealed promising results.

In summary, both fetal or maternal elements of the placenta can be considered as rich sources of stem cells as they exhibit features of both cells which are of embryonic and mesenchymal origin. They possess common characteristics of ESCs and adult MSCs and do not express any of the hematopoietic cell markers. As mentioned, P-MSCs provide an exciting research area and further investigations and clinical trials are required before they are deemed safe to be used as a treatment option for various debilitating diseases.

7.3.5 Adipose-Derived Stem Cells

As previously discussed, MSCs are non-hematopoietic cells, which are of mesodermal descent and are present in various number of organs and connective tissues. Stem cells that have similar characteristics to bone marrow–derived MSCs have been isolated from various other tissue sources present in our bodies. However, the most common problems researchers face is the low quantities of cells and limited amounts of tissues when harvested.

Most adult progenitor stem cells require some amount of ex vivo expansion before they can be used in preclinical and clinical trials to allow us to understand the safety and efficacy of these cells as standard of care. One of the types of stem cells identified are MSCs derived from adipose tissue present in our bodies. These stem cells are termed as *adipose-derived stem cells* (ASCs). The stem cells derived from adipose tissue is one of the most promising areas of research identified so far.

ASCs share many common characteristics with BM-MSCs. They are capable of extensive proliferation, possess the ability to convert into multilineage cells, and display noticeable potency both *in vitro* and *in vivo*. Adipose tissue is ubiquitous and can be easily obtained in large quantities with mild patient discomfort. Hence the use of these stem cells as both research tools and cellular therapies have proved their efficacy and safety in preclinical and clinical studies.[32]

Adipose tissue represents a vast and accessible source of adult stem cells with the potential to differentiate along multiple lineage pathways. There are at least five different types of adipose tissue that exist: mammary, white, bone marrow, mechanical, and brown.[32] Each of these serves an important distinct biological function. For example, in the bone marrow, adipose tissue serves a dual role: both a passive and active role. Brown adipose tissue is thermogenic, which means that it generates heat through the expression of unique proteins that short-circuits the mitochondrial gradient.[32] During infancy, brown tissue is found in all the major organs, but then disappears in adulthood.[32] Mammary tissue provides nutrients and energy during lactation via pregnancy hormones. Mechanical tissue provides support to the eye, hand, and other pivotal structures. Finally, white adipose tissue functions by storing energy and providing insulation to the body. The discovery of the various types of adipose stem cells has brought forth a greater appreciation of these tissues and their functional role in the body.

One of the research domains involving ASCs include wound healing. Wound healing is in an intricate and a complex process that involves well matched efforts of various types of cells and cytokines that they release. Further developments in this area has led to the understanding of how ASCs contribute to wound healing and tissue regeneration. ASCs now present various choices to clinical researchers in treating difficult wounds.

Topical administration of autologous ASCs in conjunction with type I collagen sponge matrix in murine models with diabetic ulcers has led to accelerated healing of these ulcers.[33] A clinical study conducted using human ASCs in treatment of radiation-induced tissue damage. The patients participating in this clinical study reported progressive improvement in tissue hydration and new vessel formation.[34]

ASCs also have potential application in harnessing immunomodulatory effects to treat various allergic and autoimmune diseases. A rat allergic rhinitis model was used to demonstrate the use of ASCs to treat allergic rhinitis. The rats were intravenously administered ASCs which then migrated to the surface of the nasal mucosa. Here these ASCs demonstrated inhibition of eosinophilic inflammation, modulated T-cell activity. This led to the reduction in allergic symptoms in these rat models.[35]

ASCs within the realm of possibility have proved to be effective in their potential use in regenerative medicine. They prove to offer a variety of possibilities to enhance tissue repair and tissue defects in numerous congenital diseases, cancer, and trauma.[36]

7.3.6 Embryonic Stem Cells

ESCs are derived from totipotent stem cells of early mammalian embryos. These stem cells are capable of unlimited, undifferentiated proliferation *in vitro*. ESCs possess the ability to type-match tissues for each patient. This can be accomplished either through a process known as *stem cell banking* or *using cloning*. ESCs are advantageous because they can also be maintained for long culture periods, therefore providing a great number of cells for tissues that would normally not be derived directly from a tissue source. Embryonic cells are pluripotent in nature because of the formation of a teratoma. This property reveals the capabilities of stem cells to tissue-engineer multiple tissue types and illustrates the importance of using terminally differentiated cells without latent properties. A critical step in regenerative medicine is the ability to control the differentiation of the cells to the desired tissue types. Differentiation of ESCs has been achieved using modification protocols whereby ES cells can be directed to express features of bone.[37,38] There are also indistinct steps of differentiation such as, embryoid body formation, which aids in the formation of ectodermal, endodermal, and mesodermal lines before terminal differentiation is initiated.

ESCs help provide insights in fundamental research based on early human development, causes preterm pregnancies, embryonic aging, and failure of pregnancy in elderly women. Human ES cell lines provide a dynamic system which help in identification of new molecular targets and development of novel drugs. For novel drugs, ES cells can be used *in vitro* to understand preliminary safety and potential toxicity profiles of the drug in humans. Human embryonic stem (ES) cell lines, therefore can help in the development of safer and more effective drugs for various human diseases.

ES cells also find their potential application in the field not only in the field of pharmacology but also in embryo-toxicology and toxicology. With the help of ESCs, we can gain clinically relevant insight to target organ toxicities of the drug. Another application of ESCs grown *in vitro* is that, large-scale use of these cells may reduce the need for animal testing in preclinical trials.[39]

Two clinical trials using human ESCs have been conducted for two indications: a safety trial using oligodendrocytes in spinal cord injury[40] and treatment of age-related macular degeneration. Results for phase I/II clinical trial of ESCs-derived retinal pigment epithelium for the treatment of age-related macular degeneration have showed no signs of hyperproliferation, tumorigenicity, ectopic tissue formation, or apparent[41] after 4 months.[42]

A human ESC-derived vaccine for lung cancer designed to trigger patient's immune system to attack telomerase, a protein that is expressed in almost all types of cancer. Telomerase, however is rarely expressed in normal adult cells. This vaccine is currently under development and will soon start clinical trials in patients with non-small lung cancer.[41]

7.3.7 Induced Pluripotent Stem Cells

Induced pluripotent stem cells (iPS) are stem cells that are generated using an adult cell (somatic cell) such as liver, skin, stomach, or any mature cell. These mature cells are provided with necessary genes that induce reprogramming of the mature cell. These reprogrammed cells transform into cells that possess all characteristics of ESCs, which can form cells of the embryonic lineages.

Furthermore, more recent advances in stem cell technology have led to development of iPS cells. Essentially, this technology takes differentiated cells and reprograms them back into an embryonic-like state.[43] This is done by transferring nuclear contents of cells into oocytes or by combining them with ESCs. As of now, there is still much to learn about the factors that control this reprogramming technique. What we do know is that the induction of iPS cells from mouse embryonic or adult fibroblasts are controlled by the following four factors: Oct3/4, Sox2, c-Myc, and Klf4, which was done under ESC culture conditions.[43] In the end, these iPS cells exhibited the morphology and growth properties of ESCs and expressed the same marker genes. Another important observation used subcutaneous transplantation of iPS cells into nude mice. This procedure resulted in tumors that contained a variety of tissues from the three germ layers.[43] This showed that although iPS cells can be of great use, they could also react negatively in the host. Overall, the presence of iPS cells contributed to mouse embryonic development. From all this data, we can conclude that pluripotent stem cells can be generated from fibroblasts with only the addition of a few growth factors.

iPSCs do not have any ethical constraint attached to it because they are reprogrammed using somatic cells when compared to how ESCs are derived. iPSCs, in theory can help create cell lines that can be genetically customized to a patient thereby reducing the possibility of the immune rejection of iPSCs. Another important feature of iPSCs is that they are relatively easy to create and do not require human eggs or embryos.

The world's first clinical trial was launched in Riken Centre for Developmental Biology in Kobe, Japan. Riken Center initiated the first-in-man clinical study with iPSC-derived retinal pigment epithelial (RPE) cells. Ministry of Health, Labour and Welfare, Japan provided Riken Center the green light based on the successful and rigorous *in vitro* and preclinical experiments in animals. The study was designed as an open-label and to assess the safety of autologous iPSC-derived RPE in patients who have wet age-related macular degeneration.

The following figure provides a visual representation of some of the major sources of stem cells (Figures 7.2).

7.3.8 Cell Isolation

Many biochemical experiments function by collecting large numbers of cells and then physically disturbing them to extract their inner components. If the sample happens to be a piece of tissue, composed of various types of cells, heterogeneous cell clusters will be mixed together. To obtain as much data as possible about an individual's cell type, researchers have developed methods of detaching cells from tissues and separating and organizing the various types. Thus, these controls result in a rather homogeneous population of cells that can then be evaluated. This could be done either directly following the procedure or after their number has been significantly increased by granting the cells to proliferate as a pure culture.

The first step in isolating cells from a tissue that contains a heterogeneous mixture of cell types is to disturb the extracellular matrix that holds the cells together. Cells from fetal or neonatal tissues generally produce the highest yield of viable cells. The mechanism of

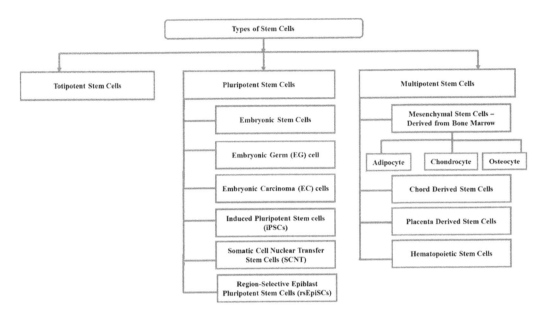

FIGURE 7.2 Cell types.

separation involves the use of proteolytic enzymes (such as trypsin and collagenase) that will digest proteins in the extracellular matrix.

One of the most practiced cell-separation techniques uses a fluorescent antibody dye that is linked to specific cells. Following the technique, the labeled cells can be separated from the unlabeled ones in a fluorescent cell sorter. In this machine, cells travel in a single file and pass through a laser beam, which measures the fluorescence of each cell. After exiting the beam, the cells are given a positive or a negative charge, depending on whether they are fluorescent; they are then diverted by a strong electric field into their appropriate container. This is a truly remarkable machine that has facilitated the use of cell culture isolation for tissue engineering.

Most eukaryotic cells stop dividing after a certain number of cell divisions in culture; this process is termed *cell senescence*. This finite amount of division is a result of the gradual shortening of the cell's telomeres. Human fibroblasts can bypass cell senescence and proliferate indefinitely by providing them with the gene that encodes telomerase; they can then proliferate as an "immortalized" cell line. However, some human cells will be unfazed by this trick because they possess checkpoints that regulate the growth of the cell. In this event, one must also inactivate the checkpoints to promote continued division.

Perhaps the most promising cell cultures to ever be developed are the human ES cell lines. These cells are from the inner cell mass of the early embryo and have the potential to proliferate indefinitely into any part of the body. The use embryonic cells could revolutionize medicine by providing cells that can repair damaged tissues.

7.3.9 Culture Conditions

Cell culture spans across diverse biological systems. Stem cells provide exciting research possibilities and potential to develop therapeutic products to treat various diseases as well as allow researchers to study how a disease develops. To develop cell lines with stem cells, we need to create appropriate culture conditions to maintain the growth and development of required stem cells.

7.3.10 Pluripotent Stem Cells

Pluripotent stem cells (PSC) include both human embryonic stem cells (hESCs) and induced pluripotent stem cells.[44] hESC lines can be derived and cultured under various conditions. These hESC lines can be used in cell transplantations, but currently these stem cells lines are used for various research purposes. Culture conditions for human PSCs share similar protocols as that of mammalian stem cells. However, to maintain human PSCs in an undifferentiated state requires additional factors that need to be taken into consideration. These additional factors allow the stem cells to maintain their characteristics of self-renewal and pluripotency.

Over the last decade or so, multiple methods of human PSCs culture techniques have evolved. Most of these techniques evolved rapidly as these specialized stem cells were found to be the solution for the current pressing needs in regenerative medicine and drug discovery. Regardless of rapid advancements in culture techniques, we still currently face multiple problems that needs to be resolved if these stem cells are to be used for future application. The challenges we face as trying to culture human PSCs include

- Lack of standardized protocols for specific applications
- An absence of efficient conditions and excessive apoptotic and spontaneous differentiation signals during cell processing
- The impurity or heterogeneity of propagated cells[45,46]
- Genomic instability related to chromosomal abnormalities[47]
- Potential tumorigenicity[48,49]

Mammalian cells that are cultured *in vitro* requires additional growth media, extracellular matrices and environmental factors.

Growth Medium: The most important factor that influences the human PSCs is growth medium. Growth medium and the conditions that are required for the culture of human PSCs have undergone a dynamic change since they were used for hESC culture.[50] First-generation human ESC growth medium contained fetal bovine serum (FBS) and undefined secretory components from mouse embryonic fibroblasts (MEFs). However, recent trends indicate standardized and better-defined growth medium which do not contain any xenogeneic elements.[51,52] Chemical mediums which are serum-free, xeno-free may be more suitable for culturing a broad range of human ESCs and human iPSCs.

Extracellular Components: Extracellular components used for culture of stem cells include a diverse range of organic matrices from animal cells, hydrogel, individual matrix proteins, synthetic surfaces, and a few commercially available xenogeneic-free components.

Extracellular matrix proteins (ECM): These ECM proteins are developmentally regulated and provide the framework that can support human PSCs self-renewal capabilities.[53] Unfortunately, use of ECM for maintenance and expansion of human PSC is limited because the high cost of obtaining highly purified proteins.

Synthetic Surfaces: These surfaces when part of the culture medium, mimic major signal transduction pathways that are required for human PSC growth.

Environmental Cues: These cues are both physical and physiological environments that encourage hESCs growth, temperature, humidity, osmosity, acidity, rigidity of growth surfaces, cell density, gas diffusion exchange, modes of multicellular associations etc.

These factors need to be taken into consideration when defining the culture conditions for culturing human ESC and human iPSC cell lines.

7.3.11 Mesenchymal Stem Cells

MSCs are multipotent stem cells that reside mostly in the bone marrow. They are capable of differentiating *in vitro* and *in vivo* into cell of the bone, cartilage, and cardiac and skeletal muscle. They exhibit a unique *in vitro* expansion.

Many studies that involve the use of MSCs require large numbers of them. Despite the need for large number of cells, only a limited amount of information on optimization of culture conditions are available. Currently lot of inconsistencies are present concerning the media conditions, the starting and passaging cell-plating density, the culture surfaces, and the addition of supplementary factors for the successful isolation and expansion of MSCs that ends up with heterogeneous cell populations both in *in vitro* experiments and in clinical trials.[54]

MSCs culture conditions involve the use of animal-derived growth supplements such a fetal bovine serum, which may lead to complications when used during clinical trials to grow them. When MSCs need to be used for clinical purposes, culture media should be devoid of all animal derived growth supplements and products.

7.4 PRIMARY CELLS

A primary cell is defined as a cell taken directly from a living organism and established for growth *in vitro*. These cells are representative of the main tissue from which they have been isolated. Compared to cell lines, primary cells are not immortalized, meaning they have a finite viability. Usually these cells can be manipulated in cell culture for a limited time after which they either senesce or die or become transformed and can no longer be considered primary cells.

Cultures prepared directly from a tissue without cell proliferation are termed *primary cultures*. These can be formed with or without the initial step that is needed to separate the different cells. Cells in primary cultures can be extracted from the primary culture dish and later be induced to proliferate into a larger number of secondary cultures. With this technique, the cells may be repeatedly cultured for a long period. Primary cells often display differentiated properties that are appropriate to their origin. For instance, fibroblasts continue to secrete collagen and cells derived from skeletal muscle fuse to form muscle fibers that contract spontaneously in the culture. Because these attributes only occur in culture, it is often difficult to study them within intact tissues.

7.4.1 Characteristics of Primary Cells

There are several properties of primary cells that distinguish them from the properties associated with cell lines. First, primary cells have a finite life span. Primary cells are taken directly from a living organism, which means that they will eventually die, as do our cells over time. Primary cells can be quite diverse and have also demonstrated that they can change in culture. For this reason, it is encouraged to conduct primary cell experiments as soon as possible. Another important characteristic to note is that these cells are not immortalized. There is no modification or alteration associated with these cells; they are what they are. Finally, unlike cell lines, primary cells tend to be much less stable in culture and more difficult to control. Both cell lines and primary cells present a unique array of characteristics that can be used in research.

7.5 CELL LINES

7.5.1 Cell Lines

For studies involving use of cell lines, immortalized cell lines are convenient because they can be maintained as a cell line in cell culture over a long period. Primary cell lines, on the other hand, are not well characterized, have a limited shelf life, and are notoriously slow in growing. However, there is a distinct advantage in using primary cells for tissue engineering and that is safety. Established cell lines by the time they have become established are generally considered to be unsafe for *in vivo* use because there is the possibility of "uncontrolled growth" once transplanted *in vivo*. On the other hand, primary cells being considered for *in vivo* use are free from adventitious infectious agents and have been cultured in compatible media for tissue-engineering purposes that involve transplantation of these cells into humans. This is not to say that cell lines can never be or should not be used for tissue engineering purposes. Even today cell lines remain as excellent tools for *in vitro* research experiments, but they are not recommended for *in vivo* trials in patients. There is a burgeoning interest in the use of iPSCs and cells derived from ESCs. These would be the "new generation" of cell lines as opposed to the standard cell lines used in biological research that have been established in cell culture over many decades. Although the safety issues with the use of the "new generation" cell lines are still being debated, it is widely accepted that they should be considered for *in vivo* purposes. Currently, most of the *in vivo* data being generated report on the use of adult stem cells including BM-MSCs, adipose-derived MSCs, and placenta- and cord-blood–derived adherent stem cells.

7.5.2 Complications of Cell Lines

There is a chance that some human cell lines can carry pathogens, which can pose as a potential health hazard to lab workers. Moreover, they can also become contaminated with other microorganisms such as, bacteria, fungi, or viruses, which may spread to other cell lines. If the cells are to be used for animal experiments, either as grafts or to derive tumors, it is critical that they are free of pathogens. As mentioned before, cell lines can be propagated in culture indefinitely and may be pre-transformed, meaning that they can be unpredictable and perhaps even risky to work with. It is advisable to use primary cells when planning clinical applications because cell lines have the potential of going rogue and causing serious adverse events. For the most part, cell lines are mostly appropriate for basic research.

Up until this point, we have introduced some of the fundamental aspects of tissue biology and the pros and cons of using primary cells versus cell lines. Although primary cells as well as cell lines are all excellent candidates for tissue engineering, there is a major problem: cells are dynamic living things. For the most part, cells are obtained from other non-self sources. This can often stimulate an immune response in the recipient in which the immune system rejects the transplanted cells and may lead to serious complications. In the following section, we will discuss the biology of cell rejection and the outcomes that are associated with it.

7.6 BIOLOGY OF CELL REJECTION

Traditionally, bone marrow transplantation has been the most instructive in guiding immune rejection of human cells taken from donors and introduced into recipients. Cells may be obtained from identical donors where donor cells pose no rejection threat from the recipient; cells may be obtained from siblings or parents as donors but are matched for HLA subtypes and other markers; cells may be obtained from unrelated donors and again matched for HLA markers.

Normally, when the host accepts a successful transplant, the body reacts by revascularizing the incoming graft. On the other hand, the body can reject the transplant if the graft is unsuccessful. In this event, inflammatory mediators rush to the site of transplant and release a plethora of signals, which convey messages to other cells of the body. Currently, immunosuppressive therapy and immune tolerance are two pivotal strategies used to increase transplant survival and function in the host.

The adaptive immune system is responsible for the immune response that leads to rejection after transplantation. Xenografts are grafts that are performed between members of different species. They have the most disparity because they undergo swift immune response, which leads to rejection. On the other hand, allografts are grafts that are performed between members of the same species who vary genetically. This is the most common form of transplantation. Because of an array of genetic differences present between species, the immune system elicits a response that leads to immune rejection of allografts and xenografts.

7.6.1 Immunobiology of Rejection

7.6.1.1 Genetic Background

Histocompatibility antigens responsible for the most vigorous allograft rejection reactions are located on the major histocompatibility complex (MHC). They are inherited as haplotypes or two half sets (one from each parent). This makes a person half identical to each of his or her parents with respect to the MHC complex. Every person expresses 6 MHC1 alleles (HLA-A, HLA-B, HLA-C—one from each parent) and at least 6 MHC2 alleles (HLA-DQ, HLA-DP, HLA-DR—one from each parent). The MHC molecules are divided into two classes. The class I molecules are normally expressed on all nucleated cells, whereas the class II molecules are expressed only on the professional antigen-presenting cells (APCs), such as dendritic cells, activated macrophages, and B cells. The physiological function of the MHC molecules is to present antigenic peptides to T cells. The class I molecules are responsible for presenting antigenic peptides from within the cell (e.g., antigens from the intracellular viruses, tumor antigens, self-antigens) to CD8 T cells. The class II molecules present extracellular antigens such as extracellular bacteria to CD4 T cells. The activation of T cells is dependent on two essential signals. In addition to the bond formed by the MHC and the TCR, there is also the need for a secondary co-stimulatory response. This secondary response occurs when a bond is formed between the molecule B7 and CD28 on APCs and Helper T cells, respectively.

7.6.2 Mechanisms of Rejection

The immune response to a transplanted organ consists of both cellular (lymphocyte mediated) and humoral (antibody mediated) mechanisms. The rejection reaction consists of the sensitization stage and the effector stage.

7.6.2.1 Sensitization Stage

In this stage, the CD4 and CD8 T cells, via their T-cell receptors, recognize the alloantigens expressed on the cells of the foreign graft. Two signals are needed for recognition of an antigen; the first is provided by the interaction of the T cell receptor with the antigen presented by MHC molecules, the second by a costimulatory receptor/ligand interaction on the T cell/APC surface.

7.6.2.2 Effector Stage

Initially, nonimmunologic "injury responses" (ischemia) induce a nonspecific inflammatory response. After activation, CD4-positive T cells initiate macrophage-mediated delayed type hypersensitivity (DTH) responses and provide help to B cells for antibody production. Endothelial cells activated by T cell-derived cytokines and macrophages express class II MHC, adhesion molecules, and costimulatory molecules. Following sensitization stage, the effector stage uses either direct or indirect pathway to convey messages to the immune system.

7.6.2.3 Direct Pathway

In the direct pathway, host T cells recognize intact allo-MHC molecules on the surface of the donor or stimulator cell. This pathway is presumably the dominant pathway involved in the early alloimmune response. When the dendritic cells are introduced, they migrate out of the graft and travel into the draining lymph nodes where they present their alloantigens to the host T cells. In the end, this pathway generates cytotoxic T lymphocytes (CTLs) that will directly lyse the graft cells.

7.6.2.4 Indirect Pathway

Essentially, in the indirect pathway, the donor MHC molecule is ingested by the recipient dendritic cells, which then derive a peptide from that allogenic MHC molecule. This foreign peptide is the presented by self-DCs to the T cells and then performs an appropriate immune response.

7.6.3 Role of Natural Killer Cells

The natural killer (NK) cells are important in transplantation because of their ability to distinguish allogenic cells from self and their potent cytolytic effector mechanisms. Unlike T and B cells, NK cells are activated by the absence of MHC molecules on the surface of target cells ("missing self" hypothesis). Recent studies have indicated that NK cells are present and activated following infiltration into solid organ allografts. NK cell inactivation or depletion also harbors the promise that it may improve the long-term outcome of transplanted organs.

7.6.4 Clinical Stages of Rejection

7.6.4.1 Hyper-Acute Rejection

In hyper-acute rejection, the transplanted tissue is rejected within minutes to hours because vascularization is rapidly destroyed. Hyper-acute rejection is humorally mediated by B cells and occurs because the recipient has preexisting antibodies against the graft, which can be induced by prior blood transfusions, multiple pregnancies, prior transplantation, or xenografts against which humans already have antibodies.

7.6.4.2 Acute Rejection

Acute rejection manifests commonly in the first 6 months after transplantation. Unlike hyper-acute rejection, acute rejection is primarily cell mediated by T cells. These T cells can either be cytotoxic T cells, which directly destroy the graft or they can be helper T cells, which behave differently by recruiting cytokines and promoting inflammation.

7.6.4.3 Humoral Rejection

Humoral rejection is form of allograft injury and subsequent dysfunction, primarily mediated by antibody and complement. It can occur immediately after transplantation (hyperacute) or during the first week. The antibodies are either preformed antibodies or represent anti-donor antibodies that develop after transplantation.

7.6.4.4 Chronic Rejection

Chronic rejection develops months to years after acute rejection episodes have subsided. Chronic rejections are both antibody- and cell-mediated. Chronic rejection appears as fibrosis and scarring in all transplanted organs, but the specific histopathological picture depends on the organ transplanted. The following table shows the risk factors associated with chronic rejection (Figures 7.3).

1. Previous episode of acute rejection
2. Inadequate immunosuppression
3. Initial delayed graft function
4. Donor-related factors
5. Reperfusion injury to organ
6. Long cold ischemia time
7. Recipient-related factors
8. Post transplant infection

FIGURE 7.3   Risk factors of chronic rejection.

7.6.5 Transplant Tolerance and Minimizing Rejection

Rejection cannot be completely prevented; however, a degree of immune tolerance to the transplant does develop. Tissue typing or cross-matching is performed prior to transplantation to assess donor-recipient compatibility for human leukocyte antigen (HLA) and ABO blood group and to ensure the safety of the procedure. There are several tests that can be executed. In one of the first tests, the ABO blood group compatibility is tested because incompatibility between the blood groups leads to rapid rejection. As always, it is important to monitor the patients with proper immunosuppressive treatment. Lastly, mixed lymphocyte reaction (MLR) can be used to assess the degree of MHC class I and class II compatibility. However, it is not a rapid test and can be used only in cases involving living related donors. It is rarely used at present.

7.6.6 Prevention and Treatment of Graft Rejection

Essentially, prevention and treatment are two main goals of immunosuppressive therapy. Drugs are designed to inhibit T cell activation and effector functions. However, one important issue with drugs is that they provide non-specific immunosuppression, and thus patients become more susceptible to infections (especially to intracellular microbes) and also have increased incidence of cancer. This is because of the depletion of circulating lymphocytes in the body. More specifically, when dealing with cancers such as leukemia, hematopoietic stem cell transplantation can be performed. The first step is to ablate the existing bone marrow to create room for the recipient cells. This causes a deficiency in erythrocytes and B-cell lymphocytes. This makes the person temporarily vulnerable because of their severely compromised immune system. It is critical to monitor the patient for the time being until the transplant is accepted.

7.6.7 Graft-versus-Host Disease and Bone Marrow Transplantation

When discussing bone marrow transplants, it is crucial to address the pathophysiological effects associated with graft-versus-host disease (GVHD). After a transplant, cytotoxic T cells will attempt to destroy the host. In most transplants, this is not life-threatening because of the increased number of host lymphocytes that are recruited in response to the graft. However, GVHD can be life-threatening if the host lacks the appropriate immune response to the grafted cells. For marrow transplants, this is usually the case because recipients either have an immunodeficiency or have been irradiated to ablate the marrow in an attempt to eradicate the cancer.

7.6.8 Immunosuppressive Agents

There are several different classes of drugs that are used in immunosuppression therapy. These drugs are coordinated into two phases. First is the initial induction phase, which requires much higher doses of these drugs, and second is the later maintenance phase, which requires lower dose, but is used for a longer period of time. A summary of the classes of drugs and their mechanisms of action can be found in Figure 7.4.

7.6.9 Antibodies

In addition to the various therapeutic agents, there are also two antibodies IL-2 receptor antagonist drugs. Specifically, these drugs are basiliximab and daclizumab, which are FDA-approved monoclonal antibodies used for kidney transplantation induction. Antithymocyte globulins are another class of monoclonal antibodies that are also used for treatment. These are derived from either equine or rabbit sources and are approved for the treatment of rejection. They also have been used as induction agents at some transplantation centers. They function by binding and depleting the T cells by inducing phagocytosis or complement-mediated lysis. Essentially, antibodies interact with lymphocyte surface antigens, depleting circulating thymus-derived lymphocytes and interfering with cell-mediated and humoral immune responses. Adverse effects such as fever, chills, thrombocytopenia, leukopenia, and headache typically occur with the first few doses.

Now that we understand the immune system responds to these cells, we can now introduce the next section of this chapter. The next step is to understand how these cells can be stimulated and influenced in a clinical setting. Cells can be induced in a variety of ways through an assortment of energy sources and growth factors.

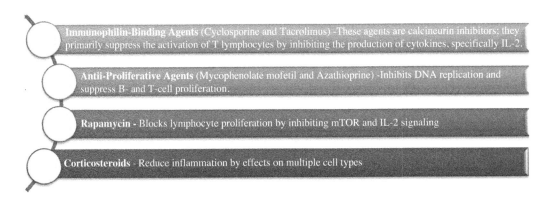

FIGURE 7.4 Therapeutic agents and their mechanisms of action.

7.6.10 Immunomodulation by Mesenchymal Stem Cells

MSCs have found to be useful in alleviating various immune disorders because of their ability to control immune responses. In patients receiving bone marrow transplants, a common issue that occurs is the GvHD. MSCs have successfully been used in these cases to reverse GvHD,[55,56] especially in patients with severe steroid resistance.[57-59]

Likewise, in patients suffering from systemic lupus erythematosus (SLE) and Chron's disease, autologous and allogenic MSCs used could reduce inflammation of the bowel and damage to the kidneys. This was possible because of the induction of regulatory T cells in these patients[(43-46)]. Recent research indicates that BM-MSCs have known to improve multiple system atrophy (MSA), multiple sclerosis (MS), amyotrophic lateral sclerosis (ALS),[60-62] and stroke.

Osiris Prochymal became the first stem cell drug to be approved by FDA in 2012 to treat GvHD and Crohn's disease.

As mentioned previously, MSCs have known to possess immunomodulation properties and are effective in treating various immune system related disorders. Both *in vivo* and *in vitro* studies indicated that, MSCs own the ability to suppress excessive immune responses of T cells, B cells, dendritic cells, macrophages, and NK cells.[63,64] Speculation exists that MSCs can regulate immune response with a collective effect of many immunosuppressive mediators.

Even with extensive research that is being conducted in trying to understand the immunomodulation ability of MSCs, we are far from developing a mature clinical technology to use the same in extensive real-life applications as standard of care. MSCs are free of ethical issues, can be derived from various sources, have low immunogenicity, and there is no risk of teratomas. This versatility of MSCs enables them to be used in current clinical applications. However, their widespread use as standard of care is still questionable.

7.7 GROWTH FACTORS

7.7.1 What Are Growth Factors?

Growth factors are critical signaling molecules that instruct cells. It is possible to achieve tissue regeneration in patients by enabling control over growth factor delivery. Simply put, growth factors can be ordinary hormones or proteins that elicit a specific physiologic function. There is an enormous amount of different growth hormones and proteins that are responsible for monitoring appropriate development. The same growth factor can generate different responses depending on the type of cell receptors that it binds to. This creates a scenario in which growth factors can ultimately control every metabolic function in the body. Let us now examine some of the specific growth factors and their mechanisms of action.

In general, growth factors do not act in an endocrine fashion. Instead, they exhibit short-range diffusion and act locally because of their short half-lives. For example, VEGF has a half-life of less than 30 minutes when infused intravenously.[65] To reiterate, the ability of a growth factor to deliver a signal to a distinct population of cells is not exclusively determined by its own identity or its ability to diffuse through the extracellular matrices.

The types of receptors that receive the signal also play an equal role in the function of the growth factor. Growth factors are very effective because of their soluble nature and can elicit cellular responses in a biological environment far removed from its original site of synthesis and secretion.[66] The specific cellular response trigged by growth factor signaling can result in a wide range of cellular actions, including cell survival, and migration, differentiation or proliferation of a specific subset of cells. A complex array of events must first occur before the signal can be transduced into the cell nucleus. These events involve cytoskeleton protein phosphorylation, ion fluxes, gene expression, protein synthesis, and an eventual biological response.[67]

7.7.2 Common Growth Factors Used in Tissue Engineering

Some of the currently used growth factors involved in tissue regeneration include: angiopoietin, basic fibroblast growth factor (bFGF), bone morphogenetic protein (BMP), epidermal growth factor (EGF), fibroblast growth factor (FGF), hepatocyte growth factor (HGF), insulin-like growth factor (IGH), nerve growth factor (NGF), platelet-derived growth factor (PDGF), transforming growth factor (TGF), vascular endothelial growth factor (VEGF; Figure 7.5).

It is important to note that the use of large quantities of VEGF may be detrimental because it could lead to unwanted vessel formation at non-target sites, such as dormant tumors. Usually, the infusion of certain factors lack specific cell population targets and therefore could result in an inadequate biological response. Thus, it is important to carefully deliver these factors to the target sites and then continue to closely monitor them for any abnormal behavior.

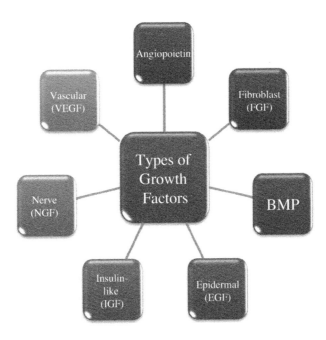

FIGURE 7.5   Growth factors.

The first step in angiogenesis requires VEGF, FGF, and angiopoietin-2 to be administered together. This disrupts the structure of the existing blood vessels and promotes proliferation and migration of new cells to the site to generate new vessels. Angiopoietin-1 and PDGF-BB then stabilize these newly formed blood vessels.[68] This example illustrates the importance of using the appropriate growth factors and the timing of administration at the desired site.

7.7.3 Growth Factor Delivery

The encapsulation process of growth factors for their controlled release is a critical strategy for growth factor delivery in tissue engineering. Its relative simplicity can provide a better alternative to chemical conjugation. Factor delivery can be combined with other variables of scaffolds to provide tissue interactions and elicit a wanted cellular response. Materials that are injected or transplanted can be readily fabricated and engineered to possess mechanical strength, porosity, and appropriate degradation rates, making them great vessels for growth factor delivery. Some physical methods of growth factor encapsulation are solvent casting, freeze-drying, melt-molding, phase emulsion, and gas foaming.[69]

Combining various methods is often used to bypass limitations. For example, a high initial release of growth factor can be easily accomplished through various techniques. However, by encapsulating the growth factors in a solvent cast and a gas foaming scaffold, you can significantly increase the potency of the growth factors and sustain a longer release of these growth factors at the target site. The area of the material that is encapsulating the growth factor will generally determine at what diffusion rate the growth factors are presented. Up until this point, a variety of techniques to combine growth factors with natural or synthetic materials and chemicals have been developed. These factors will be available to cells that encounter the matrix and thus control cell fate through localized signals.[70,71]

7.7.4 Therapeutic Uses of Hematopoietic Growth Factors

Before going into the clinical uses of hematopoietic growth factors, it may be useful to understand their biological actions. These factors are a class of growth factors that are responsible for the growth of blood cells and bone marrow proliferation. These hematopoietic growth factors are a diverse set of hormones with effects on hematopoietic lineages at various points in their developmental cycle.[72] So far, they have entered clinical trials and have displayed encouraging results clinical situations. Currently, phase II and III clinical trials are trying to use these factors, either alone or in combinations, to modify disease states and to eradicate many of the side effects associated with other therapeutic agents, such as cytotoxic anticancer agents.[72] Many other disease states can also be treated with these growth factors in a similar fashion. Not all hematopoietic growth factors have been studied in humans thus far. However, they show great promise because of the positive results provided from the other related growth factors. Some of these factors are used to clinically mobilize peripheral blood stem cells prior to harvesting the stem cells for transplantation (e.g., granulocyte colony-stimulating factor [GCSF] either alone or in combination with granulocyte macrophage colony-stimulating factor [GMCSF] is used to mobilize CD34+ peripheral blood stem cells).

From this section, we can appreciate the significant impact of biological stimulation using growth factors. It is no wonder that this field of study has become a prominent area of regenerative medicine. The use of these growth factors is limitless because for every type of tissue in the body, there is a respective growth factor that works to control the metabolic function of that specific organ. These growth factors can also target other types of cells and elicit different responses as well. Tissue engineering focuses on the most critical factors and hormones and manipulates them in a way in which a positive result can occur. So far, several clinical trials associated with growth factors have been carried out and many have shown promising results. In the following section, we will turn our attention to the uses of stem cells in tissue engineering and build on the different kinds of stimuli associated with physical interaction.

7.8 USE OF STEM CELLS IN TISSUE ENGINEERING

7.8.1 Introduction

Up until now, the gold standard for replacing damaged organs has been through organ transplantation. Unfortunately, year after year, there is a shortage of organs and tissues that can be transplanted because of the aging population. Therefore, researchers are constantly trying to develop new ways to harvest and create organs to those in need. Scientists have applied the principles of cell transplantation with tissue engineering to achieve this alternative. The field of tissue engineering has opened many doors for cellular therapy. In this section, we will discuss some of the applications and technologies that are being used for the engineering of tissues and organs.

The main goal of tissue engineering is to repair organ pathologies. It is based upon the foundations of cell transplantation and materials science. Tissue engineering uses scaffolds to fill the tissue void and provide structural support. Tissue engineering can be envisioned in two different ways. *In vivo* experiments operate by stimulating the body's own regeneration response with the appropriate materials. On the other hand, ex vivo experiments function by expanding cells in culture. The cells acquired for these experiments can come from different sources. Autologous cells are preferred because they will not evoke an immunologic response and thus the side effects of immunosuppressive agents can be avoided.

Although autologous cells are recognized as the ideal transplantation resource, many patients with end-stage diseases are unable to provide sufficient cells for transplantation. Therefore, stem cells are an alternate source of cells for the formation of the desired tissue. hESCs can be derived from discarded embryos and have the advantage of being able to self-renew indefinitely. However, these represent an allogeneic resource and thus their use would require high-dose immunosuppressant therapy.

To circumvent immune rejection and the use of high-dose immunotherapy, new stem cell technologies such as somatic cell nuclear transfer and parthenogenesis have been developed. These procedures offer an alternative route to create a vast supply of ESC that can differentiate into any cell type, while not being rejected by the patient's immune system. Although many tissues have been created with ESC, they are not used clinically because of an inability to control differentiation. It is difficult to control them because of their ability to form multiple tissue types. In the meantime, the advancement of new genomics and bioinformatics technologies continues to offer new insights into the understanding and control of ESC growth and differentiation and their application to engineering tissues. Soon, these new technologies will allow for the generation of an unlimited supply of any cell type in the body.

7.8.2 Stem Cells

Ever since the discovery of stem cells, there has always been much controversy surrounding the ethical and political principles of embryos in research experiments.[50] hESCs are obtained from the inner cell mass of a blastocyst using an immunosurgical technique. ESCs are an excellent resource for tissue engineering, given the fact that most cells cannot be expanded ex vivo. The ability of ESCs to self-renew indefinitely and differentiate into all three germ layers makes them ideal candidates for tissue engineering.

Citing ethical concerns, scientists have been working to modify the use of HESC in research trials. It is estimated that there are 400,000 frozen embryos currently in storage.[73] However, only a tiny fraction of these embryos will pose as viable products for the development of HESC lines. In the end, there is always a chance that the host's immune system can reject these successfully derived stem cells when they are implanted. This make the process very challenging and demands the development of newer technologies with higher efficacies.

7.8.3 Scaffolding Techniques

There are two main techniques that are used with scaffolding to produce engineered tissue. Scaffolding can be used as a support device in which cells are encouraged to lay down matrix to produce the foundations of a tissue for transplantation.[74] The second approach uses the scaffold as a growth factor delivery device. This strategy requires that the scaffold be combined with growth factors, by doing so, implanted cells are recruited to the scaffold site and form tissue upon and throughout the matrices.[74] The way a cell type and a scaffold are combined should be meticulously matched. It has been demonstrated that composition and architecture of scaffolds can interact and influence cell behavior. Different levels of topography have also been demonstrated to influence the cell behavior by modifying the cytoskeleton arrangements.

7.8.4 Cell Sources

The formation of engineered tissue *in vitro* requires the use of cells to fill matrices and produce matrices that resemble the native tissues. Primary cells have been the most successful source of cells. These cells are taken from patients and then used together with scaffolds to generate tissue for implantation. However, the invasive nature of cells and the potential for cells to be in a diseased state limits the effectiveness of primary cells from patient sources. Therefore, the use of stem cells, including ESCs, BM-MSCSs, and umbilical cord-derived MSCs, has attracted attention because they can avoid these limitations.

7.8.5 Somatic Cell Nuclear Transfer (Therapeutic Cloning)

Somatic cell nuclear transfer (SCNT) is an important player when it comes to tissue engineering. The mechanism of this process entails the removal of an oocyte nucleus following its replacement with a nucleus from a somatic cell obtained from a patient.[75] Chemical activation and electrical shock stimulates cell division of the oocyte up until the blastocyst stage at which time the inner cell mass is isolated and cultured. The development ceases and does not continue because the blastocyst is not transplanted back into the uterus. No sperm are used in the process; so therefore, there is no fertilization either.[75] As mentioned before, the goal of SCNT and parthenogenesis is to avoid the use of any immunosuppressants. The resulting ESCs are perfectly tailored to the patient's immune system and no immunosuppressants would therefore be required to prevent rejection.

Unfortunately, the use of cloning technology has been banned in many countries. This is because there is debate surrounding the ethical principles guiding therapeutic and reproductive cloning. However, it is still important to note and understand the critical distinction between the two. Reproductive cloning is used to create an embryo that is identical to the original cell. The cell is then implanted back into the uterus and then has the potential to give rise to an infant that is a clone of the donor.[76,77] Similarly, therapeutic cloning is also used to create identical genetic material but limited to generating only ESC lines. These ESCs possess the ability to become any type of cell, which is extremely useful when replacing any tissues or organs.[78] Studies have shown that about 3,000 people die daily of diseases that could have been treated with stem cell technology.[79] Current allogenic transplantation is somewhat problematic because of the risk of rejection by the host immune system. The use of therapeutic cloning could save countless lives because the cells are genetically identical, and it avoids the use of any immunosuppressive therapy.[80]

7.8.6 Parthenogenesis

Parthenogenesis is another procedure that requires stem cells for tissue engineering. Essentially, parthenogenesis is the creation of an offspring by a female with no contribution from the male. The stem cells that are extracted for this procedure assume the morphology and functional behavior of HESC and indicate appropriate ESC markers.[75] These markers have embryonic-like replicative ability and have been propagated *in vitro* in an undifferentiated state. Furthermore, *in vitro*, they have been differentiated into many cell types, such as cardiomyocyte-like cells, smooth muscle, adipocytes, beating ciliated epithelia, several types of epithelial cells, as well as neurons.[75] Once again, this shows the great extent to which these ESCs can differentiate into and thus be critical assets in tissue engineering.

7.8.7 Stem Cell Genomics

Although the use of stem cells has significant benefits, the pluripotency of stem cells, however, is their limitation and explains why it is difficult to control them. The ESCs possess the ability to differentiate into many cells, but the efficiency can be quite limited for certain cell types.

Genomics-guided tissue engineering is another technology that is in development. This technology works by performing microarrays during the differentiation of stem cells.[81] There have been several discoveries, which have identified numerous targets such as receptors and ligands that are used to improve the quality and quantity of differentiation. Ultimately, this technology can provide new insight into the type of neuronal cells that may be formed, but it offers clues into what our stem cell-derived neurons might be missing. With this knowledge, we can then go back to the culture system and target these specific signaling pathways. Further study of stem cell genomics will give us an understanding of its pluripotency. Eventually, it might be possible to differentiate a somatic cell into an intermediate stage, which could then be expanded and transplanted back into the patient.[75] Currently, there is much research on the genetic signature of stem cell pluripotency that has been analyzed from the gene of primate stem cells.

Experimental efforts are currently underway involving virtually every type of tissue and organ of the human body. Various tissues are at different stages of development with some already being used clinically, a few in preclinical trials, and some in the discovery stage. Recent progress suggests that engineered tissues may have an expanded clinical applicability in the future and may represent a viable therapeutic option for those who require tissue replacement or repair.

7.9 USE OF STIMULATORY INFLUENCES IN TISSUE ENGINEERING

The use of stimulatory factors in regenerative medicine is one of the hallmarks of tissue engineering. Stimulatory influences can be electrical, thermal, or mechanical forms of stimulation. Moreover, they can also be things like growth factors, hormones, and drugs, which are all designed to promote metabolic functions in the body. In this section, we'll introduce an overview of the vast amount of stimulatory influences that are being used in therapy today. In the upcoming sections, we will take a closer look at some of these factors and their applications to tissue engineering.

So, what is the purpose of using these stimulatory factors and what role do they play in tissue engineering? One of the main reasons why research is so focused on regenerative medicine is mainly because of the simple reason that people are living longer. With medicinal and technological advances, people have been able to live longer and healthier lives. This has led to a shortage of organs for transplants and has generated an increased demand for alternative forms of treatment. The answer to this urgent need is tissue engineering.

Tissue engineering is the growth of new connective tissues, or organs, from cells to produce a fully functional organ for implantation back into the donor host. To initiate the formation of a fully functional organ or tissue, the cells need to be stimulated appropriately. Stimuli is defined as the event that elicits a specific response in cells or tissue. There are three forms of physical stimuli—mechanical, electrical, and thermal. Each possesses its own characteristics and mechanisms that make them unique.

7.9.1 MSC Stimulation

Figure 7.6 shows the types of stimuli that will be discussed. We will give an overview of the procedures in this section and then go into more detail in the following sections (Figure 7.6).

7.9.2 Electrical Stimulation

One of the greatest wonders of the body is the existence of its own personal electric field. By now, it is well accepted that cells in our body relay messages using electric impulses.

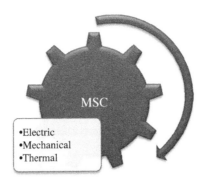

FIGURE 7.6   Physical stimulations.

Researchers have sought to investigate the topic of human electricity and how it can be applied to regenerative medicine. After extensive studies, it has been discovered that bioelectricity is inherent in wound healing. When an injury occurs, an electric field is generated. This electric field acts as a chaperone, which guides cells to the site of the wound. If the electric field is compromised, the wound would fail to heal properly. Moreover, the electrical resistivity of tissues varies frequently because the variation in tissue composition, such as tissue type, density, permeability, and electrolyte concentration. These factors combined are measured through a procedure known as the bioelectrical impedance analysis (BIA). The BIA is important because it can analyze if there are any electrical imbalances that are because of some form of nutritional or metabolic disorder. This process is great for soft tissue but remains difficult for bone tissue because of the composite material that it is made from. However, electrical measurements can still be used as excellent tools for diagnosing bone grafts during joint replacement surgery.

At the microscopic level, cells are responsive to an exogenous electric field. The discovery regarding the response of yeast[82] and diatoms[83] to electromagnetic field (EMF) stimulation was a major breakthrough because both yeast and diatoms are simple organisms, which implies that EMF occurs at even the cellular level. Furthermore, these studies also show that cell behaviors can be manipulated using external physical stimuli such as EMF.

Biological systems often respond to endogenous or exogenous electric stimulation, demonstrating that the electric field may serve as tool to control and to adjust tissue homeostasis. Till now, a variety of cells have been exposed to electric stimulation including MSCs, bone cells, and cardiac cells. Experiments have shown that the electric field influences pivotal cellular functions such as adhesion, proliferation, differentiation, and directional migration

7.9.3 Mechanical Stimulation

Articular cartilage engineering has become a rapidly growing area of research over the past decade. During this time, the field of functional tissue engineering has become widely recognized and studied. In this field, mechanical stimulations are applied to constructs to generate mechanically induced tissue. It has been known for quite some time that mechanical stimulation plays an important role in the development of healthy native cartilage.

Physical factors have become an almost essential element in tissue engineering. There are several types of mechanical loading (stimulation) involved in the direct development of tissue-engineered cartilage. Some of these include dynamic compression, fluid or tissue shear, and hydrostatic pressure. The effects of the stimulation are measured through ECM production, development of tissue functionality, and gene expression.

The goal of mechanical tissue engineering is to simply develop a viable replacement for damaged tissue. As mentioned previously, there are various types of physical stimuli that are induced when tissue is mechanically loaded. When this tissue is loaded, a signal occurs and is transported throughout cellular pathways in the body until it generates a biosynthetic response. This process is known as the mechanotransduction pathway.[84–86] With all the available research data that we have amassed, mechanical stimulation will most likely continue to remain a critical tool in tissue engineering for the years to come.

7.9.4 Thermal Stimulation

The final type of physical stimulation that we will discuss is thermal stimulation. Just as the name implies, thermal stimulation involves the use of heat to induce specific behaviors in targeted cells. After many studies, it has been concluded that during a stress response, the cell expresses a set of proteins known as *heat shock proteins*. These proteins respond to the stress signal by performing various types of physiologic functions, such as repairing damage and translocation assistance of proteins.[87] These functions can be harnessed and guided to stimulate the proliferation of MSCs. Therefore, heat shock proteins have an important influence on stem cells. In fact, studies have shown that there are some heat shock proteins that physically interact with a number of transcription factors.[87] This interaction allows the protein to have a direct influence on the cell. Alternatively, changes in the heat shock protein expression have exhibited changes in cell behavior, self-renewal potential, and differentiation.

7.9.5 Biological Stimulation

We have briefly introduced three of the major physical stimuli that are used in tissue engineering. Now, we will turn our attention to a different form of stimulation. Biological stimulants can be hormones or vitamins that display a specific role required for the stimulation of growth in living cells. For the most part, thermal, mechanical, and electrical stimuli are exogenous sources induced by some type of procedure. Endogenous stimulants are those stimulants that are produced by cells within the body. For example, cells secrete cytokines, which function as signaling molecules to either promote or inhibit tissue regeneration. Moreover, they also function by promoting or preventing adhesion, migration, differentiation, synthesis of other proteins, and many more functions. Different cells can have the same outcome or a different outcome depending on the type of cytokine that interacts with the receptors. The most pivotal signaling molecules in healing of bones and development are TGFs and BMPs. Clinically; growth factors have become common and promising in bone regeneration because of its relative simplicity and its high efficiency. Interestingly, some of these proteins can be regulated through physical stimulation as well. Often, cultured cells are introduced to both biological and physical stimuli at varying intensities.[88,89]

Some of these stimuli include electrical and electromagnetic, mechanical, laser irradiation, heat, and ultrasound. A few of these have been used in the clinic to treat defects in tissues.[90] Moreover, studies have shown that osteoblasts have shown increased proliferation and differentiation when exposed to factors like TGF and BMP.[88,91] Growth factors can be endogenously induced through the appropriate extrinsic physical stimulation.

7.9.6 Other Forms of Energy

7.9.6.1 Ultrasound Stimulation

When discussing stimulatory influences, it is almost impossible to avoid the subject of bone composition. Bone is a very dynamic material, it can break down or build up based on the metabolic requirements of our body. Usually, growth factors and hormones are the ones responsible for these catabolic/anabolic processes. However, there are many external stimulatory influences that are designed to try to mimic the physiological actions of the body. For example, therapeutic ultrasound has been used as a healing technique to treat bone fractures and avoid invasive procedures.[92] Studies have shown that ultrasound therapy has successfully been able to promote regeneration and bio-absorption.[93,94] It can treat bone defects by emitting mechanical frequencies that are above the threshold of human hearing. Ultrasound (US) therapy has been used for many years and has now become an essential tool in the clinic. High-intensity US can damage tissues; therefore, low-intensity pulsed ultrasound (LIPUS) is generally used in the clinic.

7.9.6.2 Electromagnetic Stimulation

Like electrical stimulation, electromagnetic therapy also serves a vital role in tissue engineering. One technique known as the pulsed electromagnetic field (PEMF) is routinely used when treating patients with bone defects. PEMFs method of action involves the regulation of osteoblast differentiation and proliferation.[95] This occurs when the desired cells are exposed to PEMF at a certain threshold and frequency. The pulses are intermittently induced over a period of time and the intensity of the signals is controlled to achieve the desired results. This type of therapy is commonly used in conjunction with electrical stimulation and can also be used with other physical stimuli.[95]

There are various types of stimuli that can induce a cell to perform a programmed task. There are also many other accessory stimuli that are often used in conjunction with the three main ones that we discussed. The last three sections will discuss the stimuli in greater detail including how they are being used in therapy.

7.10 ELECTRICAL STIMULATION

7.10.1 Electronic Stimulation

The cell cycle is intricate process that governs every cell in the body. Different cells have different rhythms and time frames in which they can completely go through an entire cycle. It has been shown that electrical stimulation at 448 kHz could alter and manipulate the cyclic proliferation of adipose-derived human stem cells by upregulating certain kinases.[96] This further demonstrated that capacitive resistance electro-thermal therapy (CRET) could exert an electronic stimulation and induce differentiation. There are various types of stem cell lines, however, when dealing with CRET it was best to use adipocyte stem cells for the following reasons. First, ADSC work well with CRET, and second, adipocytes can be used to discover other types of adipogenic processes.[97] During the CRET exposure, electrode pairs and a signal generator was used. Then 5-minute pulses were administered to the cells at 448 kHz. After the experiment, it was observed that the electric stimulation influenced the cell proliferation.[97] In conclusion, the 448 kHz CRET therapy is unique because it mostly uses electrical stimulation but also use mechanical and thermal stimuli at once.

It has been proven that electric currents and electric fields can influence proliferative or differentiating processes involved in tissue regeneration. Several tests, such as, flow cytometry and Western Blot have been conducted to determine the viability and differentiation potential of adipose-derived stem cells. CRET has been shown to upregulate certain proteins like PCNA and ERK1/2, which are essentials for cell proliferation.[97] Therefore, CRET could be used to stimulate proliferation of stem cells in injured tissues.

Precursor cells are also very crucial components of the regeneration process. After the cells proliferate, they will start to differentiate into their respective tissue cell types. The MSCs are a group of cells that are essential to the regeneration and are present in almost all adult tissues. These characteristics make them an excellent tool in regenerative medicine because of their capacity to self-regenerate and differentiate into different cell types. Thus, much attention has been focused on these MSCs so that they can be harvested and used in regenerative medicine.

7.10.2 Electrothermal Therapy

For many years, electronic stimulation has been used when dealing with injuries and regenerative medicine. Electrical stimulation has been shown to greatly improve regeneration of chronic injuries that were often unresponsive to any other treatment.[98] In addition, there are also many physiological benefits that have been examined using electric stimulation. For example, electrical stimulation can improve blood flow, increase elasticity of damaged tissues,[99] and reduce edema.[100] At the microscopic level, electric stimulation influences the adhesion, orientation, and migration patterns of cells.[101,102] Electric stimulation plays a pivotal role in tissue engineering because the vast amount of benefits that it has demonstrated.

Once again, CRET is a noninvasive electro-thermal therapy. It functions by releasing an electric current ranging from 400–450 kHz of radiofrequency.[103] Naturally, tissues contain an electric resistivity, thus allowing CRET currents to potentially create temperature changes in the targeted organs of therapy.[104] Furthermore, previous studies have shown that CRET stimulation at subthermal doses can induce anti-tumor and cytotoxic responses in human cancer cell lines but not in primary cells like human peripheral blood cells. These results illustrate that CRET therapy does not work alone but in cooperation with both thermal stimulation and direct electric stimulation on the cells.

7.10.3 Low-Frequency Electrical Stimulus

Low-frequency physical stimulus has also been a valuable technique that has been used to promote stem cell induction into different cell lineages. For example, *in vitro* exposure to PEMFs has been shown to exponential increase in cell proliferation.[105]

Moreover, evidence exists that the proliferative response to electric stimuli could potentially be related with cells at specific cycle phases. It has been reported that a

50 Hz frequency can induce proliferation in bone marrow stem cells by increasing the proportion of cells entering phases S and G2 of the cycle.[106] In addition, human marrow cells have also exhibited a proliferative response *in vitro* treatment when exposed to 15 Hz PEMF. Recently,[107] there have been reports that a 50 Hz exposure and a 10 Hz PEMF could both increase proliferation and block cell cycle in G1. This shows how valuable and flexible this technology is and how it can manipulate the development of cells. Furthermore, in current studies, flow cytometry has illustrated that CRET exposure can increase the number of cells in phases S, G2 and mitosis. Therefore, it can be hypothesized that therapeutic CRET can activate quiescent stem cells present in damaged tissues and thus be stimulated to enter proliferation and cell renewal that will lead to tissue repair.

As for molecular mechanisms, the mitogen-activated protein kinases (MAPK-ERK1/2) are the most significant molecules involved in transduction of proliferative signals from extracellular origin. ERK1 and ERK2 are activated through phosphorylation by MEKs (MAPK/ERK kinases). There are also other physical therapies that could promote recovery through cell proliferation by activation of ERK1/2, as seen in the US-treated human skin fibroblasts. Studies have revealed that expression of phosphorylated ERK1/2 directly increased with the amount of CRET-treated adipose-derived stem cells. This supports the claim that weak electric stimuli can activate the Ras/Raf/MEK/ERK pathways, and thus provides support to the proliferative action of CRET on human mesenchymal cells.

In conclusion, the electric stimulus used in electrothermal CRET therapy induces upregulation of the ERK1/2 signaling pathway and promotes proliferation of mesenchymal stem cells. Furthermore, an electric stimulus can be applied at a specific subthermal current to be used as a therapeutic treatment for tissue repair and regeneration.[103] CRET electrotherapy could be applied as an adjuvant to the recovery of a variety of lesions or as an alternative treatment for patients whom are sensitive to the side effects of other chemical therapies. CRET might also be useful in anti-inflammatory treatments through its ability to increase the amount of MSCs. Studies are currently underway that will investigate whether CRET could stimulate cell differentiation toward connective tissue.

7.10.4 Biomineralized Materials

In addition to CRET, the use of biomineralized biomaterials has also shown to increase the rate of osteogenic differentiation of stem cells. Biomaterials can be used as scaffolds that facilitate electrical stimulation of human mesenchymal stem cells (HMSCs), which promotes their differentiation. To test this experiment, biomineralized materials must first be planted with HMSCs. These scaffold systems contain various kinds of components to help promote stem cell differentiation.

The differentiation of the cells was shown using a biochemical assay for alkaline phosphatase (ALP) activity. As usual, ALP activity of cells cultured on control substrates is insignificant. Interestingly, ALP activity of cells cultured on the scaffolds mineralized with calcium phosphate was higher than for cells on the scaffolds mineralized with silica.[108]

Most importantly, the ALP activity of cells on the conductive biomineralized scaffolds increased the most after electrical stimulation. In the end, the analysis revealed that the nonconductive scaffolds supported differentiation of HMSCs toward osteogenic outcomes, but the application of an electrical stimulus to HMSCs further enhanced levels of ALP activity, which is a hallmark of bone tissue formation.

7.11 MECHANICAL STIMULATION

7.11.1 Introduction

We have presented evidence that mesenchymal cells are multipotent cells and can be harvested from bone marrow as well as other adult tissues. These stem cells can then develop into multiple cell lineages, ranging from fat cells to neurons. In this section, we will look at how mechanical cues can influence the fate of a MSC.

Mechanical stimulation has long been considered insignificant and has been shadowed by other types of stimuli. However, it is now evident that mechanical signals do in fact play critical roles in stem cell development. To use these signals in therapy, it is important to understand how the mechanical cues orchestrate stem cell differentiation. Only then will we be able to enhance our techniques in cell therapy and organ repair. For instance, there are various growth factors that have been used to examine the control of stem cell proliferation. HMSCs treated with fibroblast growth factor-2 resulted in an increased proliferation rate.[109] In addition, combining BMP-2 and FGF-2 further increased proliferation. This is most likely because of the synergistic effects of signal crosstalk between the two different growth factors.[110] These are just a few of the factors that are responsible for MSC proliferation. Pluripotent mesenchymal cells are ideal therapeutic targets for regenerative medicine because they can differentiate into a variety of cell types.

7.11.2 Low Magnitude Mechanical Signals

The use of low magnitude mechanical signals (LMMS) has been shown to have a twofold effect, which functions by building bone and diminishing fat in an organism. These mechanical signals indicate a potentially useful and unique therapeutic system, which could aid in tissue regeneration and repair. Moreover, these mechanical signals have been reported to show an increase in the amount of bone stem cells residing in the marrow. Furthermore, these mechanical signals favored the differentiation of the cells toward osteogenesis over adipogenesis, such that obesity was diminished and bone formation was enhanced.

After the induction of mechanical signals, MSCs have expressed various surface markers, such as Sca-1 and Pref-1.[111] The use of these markers allows us to identify MSCs. To sum it up, these factors indicate that mesenchymal cells are positively influenced by mechanical signals, which results in an increase in total number of cells.

Although potential applications of using mechanical signals are appealing, the lack of complete understanding of MSCs is evident. Further, identification of MSCs has proven to be challenging because of the difficulty in identifying these stem cells and their bordering cells with current technology.

Further studies have demonstrated that aging organisms exhibit a reduction in their stem cell count and their capacity to regenerate,[112] as well as predisposing them toward adipogenesis over osteogenesis.[113] Thus, both age and activity are important factors to consider when assessing the viability of the stem cell population.

In the end, the mechanical signals released from LMMS increase the number of progenitor cells. The ability of LMMS to deter the development of stem cells into fat could be of great use in future therapy. Likewise, the ability to orient cells toward osteogenesis would also serve as a pivotal tool in regenerative medicine.

7.11.3 Mechanical Forces

All cells in the body are in direct contact with the ECM and receive various forces from the environment under normal physiologic conditions. For example, endothelial cells undergo changes in stress and compression during stretching of muscles during muscle contractions. Knowing this basic physiology, it may be possible to use these mechanical environments to induce proliferation and differentiation of cells into specific lineages. To examine how these mechanical forces can influence cellular differentiation, we must talk a look at several approaches.

It has been demonstrated that ECM-coated magnetic beads can downregulate cell proliferation. This was shown to be as a result of a large magnetic field that exerted a twisting force upon the stem cells.[114] However, the force exerted on E-cadherin, although having no effect on cell proliferation, increased cells stiffness. What this study shows is that mechanical forces acting on E-cadherins or integrins may be able to act through different pathways to regulate embryogenesis.

Furthermore, it has been shown that compressive forces have been able to induce expression of specific transcription factors, such as Sox-9.[115] Cyclic stretching has also been applied to stem cells to investigate the effect of mechanical stress on stem cell development. Cyclic loading can enhance the differentiation of human cord–derived MSCs into osteoblast-like cells as evidenced the expression of certain markers.[116,117] Proteins ERK1/2 mediate this cyclic process and a stretch-activated channel.[117] These results suggest that mechanical stimulation can be of use in tissue engineering.

Mechanical stimuli can work in two ways. They can either work together with other soluble factors or they can work alone to regulate the fate of a stem cell. These stimulatory effects are like the native conditions that stem cells experience *in vivo*. Signals generated by mechanical stimuli mimic the cells natural environment and allow the cell to differentiate into distinct lineages. By studying these mechanical cues, we can ultimately regulate stem cell fate and behavior.

Studies mentioned previously show the various types of mechanical stimuli that act upon MSCs. Some of these include cyclic stretching, stiffness, and compressive shear stresses. There is still much research to be done before we can fully understand how to manipulate these cells, but what we do know is that these cells are superior regenerators and will be essential players in future cell-based therapy.

However, to fully understand MSCs, we must know how these cells behave *in vitro* and *in vivo* settings. As mentioned before, the release of soluble factors and cytokines govern cell behavior. Thus, by combining mechanical cues together with scaffolds and soluble factors we can form unlimited progenitor cells sources, which would enable us to design biomaterials that incorporate both chemical and physical cues that mimic the *in vivo* environment. In the end, these innovations in tissue engineering and regenerative medicine will allow us to create alternative tissues and materials to repair damaged tissues and organs with confidence and safety.

7.12 THERMAL STIMULATION

7.12.1 Introduction

In tissue engineering, the development of new procedures to differentiate cells into specific lineages via thermal, mechanical, or electrical stimuli has gained prominence. Breakthroughs in these areas would impact clinical therapy by decreasing the use of biochemical products that may have harmful side effects. Investigators are eager to discover and create innovative new procedures that would be of great value to regenerative medicine. For example, piezoelectric materials have been used to combine the stimulations of mechanical and electrical forces. Like with all research, the best way to induce a cell to differentiate *in vivo* would be to mimic its preferred environment. In this section, we will discuss some of the uses of thermal stimulation and its future role in tissue engineering.

7.12.2 Thermal Therapy

Like mechanical and electrical therapy, thermal stimulation has also shown promising results. It is used as a vital tool today in treating many diseases including osteoarthritis, a disease that affects a clear majority of elderly people. HMSC differentiation would be the best treatment, however, it takes a long time to generate desired cell populations *in vitro*.[118] Electric and mechanical therapies can catalyze the process, but not as efficiently as thermal stimulation procedures can. Studies have shown that a mild heat shock on HMSCs had a direct effect on the growth and viability of these cells.[119] In addition, the heat shock process was also able to upregulate other collagen co-factors, which demonstrated that this process could catalyze MSC differentiation.[118] This discovery serves as a pivotal stepping-stone for the collaboration between thermal technology and tissue engineering involving MSCs.

The benefits of thermal therapy are illustrated in the following example. Periodic shock was administered to osteogenic cells, which then enhanced differentiation of HMSCs.[119] This was observed by measuring the alkaline phosphatase activity and the calcium deposition in culture. Along with culture assays, immunohistochemical analyses were also conducted to get a closer look at the composition of the ECM and the type of components that were being generated.[119] Results of this study provides a strong rationale for using such stimulation in generating the appropriate cells for use as a potential treatment for patients with osteoarthritis.

In summary, it is becoming clear that thermal stimulation is an important factor in accelerating differentiation of HMSCs. Previously, it has been known that mechanical and electrical stimuli could not catalyze the differentiation process in the same way thermal therapy could do. Moreover, the intensity, interval, and duration of the heat stimulation can be further optimized and controlled to achieve differentiation in HMSCs. It is essential to continue to carry out *in vitro* and *in vivo* experiments because they will be able to give us an outlook as to how to manipulate the maturation of HMSC at different thermal doses.

7.12.3 Heat Shock Therapy

The main goal of heat shock stimulation therapy is to promote and enhance differentiation in MSCs and other co-factors necessary for maturation of cells. It has been known for some time, that when heat therapy is applied to diseased joints, it directly stimulates the activity of various cells such as chondrocytes, osteoblasts, and progenitor cells. Moreover, studies have also shown that a slight change in temperature (1.5°C–3°C above body temperature) has stimulated embryonic development and growth.[120,121]

Essentially, heat shock therapy works by promoting late osteogenic genes and diminishing the early genes. It can function this way because of the elevated ALP activity and calcium deposition, which are products of direct thermal stimulation. Furthermore, thermal stimulation allows us to enter the late stages of osteogenesis via proteins such as Runx2 and BMP2[122] This results in an enhanced mineralization. Basically, the point of thermal stimulation and heat shock therapy is to encourage the late stages of cell differentiation. At this point, the stimuli can influence and manipulate the cells behavior to produce an enhanced response.

QUESTIONS

1. Why is thermal stimulation effective?

2. In what ways do mechanical strains alter cellular behavior?

3. What are the differences between totipotent, pluripotent, and multipotent stem cells?

4. How is an iPSC different from an MSC?

5. Name three stem cell sources.

6. What are growth factors?

7. Name four growth factors commonly used in tissue engineering. What do they do?

8. How are primary cells different from cell lines?

9. Name three types of pluripotent stem cells.

10. How can graft rejection be minimized?

REFERENCES

1. De Miguel MP, Arnalich Montiel F et al. Epiblast-derived stem cells in embryonic and adult tissues. *International Journal of Developmental Biology*. 2009 53(8–10):1529–1540.
2. Chung YG, Eum JH et al. Human somatic cell nuclear transfer using adult cells. *Cell Stem Cell*. 2014 14(6):777–780.
3. Wu J, Okamura D et al. An alternative pluripotent state confers interspecies chimaeric competency. *Nature*. 2015 521(7552):316–321.

4. Friedenstein A, Friedenstein AJ et al. Osteogenesis in transplants of bone marrow cells. *Development.* 1966 16(3):381.
5. Pittenger MF, Mackay AM et al. Multilineage potential of adult human mesenchymal stem cells. *Science.* 1999 284(5411):143–147.
6. Bruder SP, Kurth AA et al. Bone regeneration by implantation of purified, culture-expanded human mesenchymal stem cells. *Journal of Orthopaedic Research.* 1998 16(2):155–162.
7. Howard D, Partridge K et al. Immunoselection and adenoviral genetic modulation of human osteoprogenitors: In vivo bone formation on PLA scaffold. *Biochemical and Biophysical Research Communications.* 2002 299(2):208–215.
8. Angel MJ, Sgaglione NA et al. Clinical applications of bioactive factors in sports medicine: Current concepts and future trends. *Sports Medicine and Arthroscopy Review.* 2006 14(3):138–145.
9. Ashton BA, Allen TD et al. Formation of bone and cartilage by marrow stromal cells in diffusion chambers in vivo. *Clinical Orthopaedics and Related Research.* 1980 294–307.
10. Majumdar MK, Banks V et al. Isolation, characterization, and chondrogenic potential of human bone marrow-derived multipotential stromal cells. *Journal of Cellular Physiology.* 2000 185(1):98–106.
11. Haynesworth SE, Barer MA et al. Cell surface antigens on human marrow-derived mesenchymal cells are detected by monoclonal antibodies. *Bone.* 1992 13(1):69–80.
12. Tilley S, Bolland BJRF et al. Taking tissue-engineering principles into theater: Augmentation of impacted allograft with human bone marrow stromal cells. *Regenerative Medicine.* 2006 1(5):685–692.
13. McElreavey KD, Irvine AI et al. Isolation, culture and characterisation of fibroblast-like cells derived from the Wharton's jelly portion of human umbilical cord. *Biochemical Society Transactions.* 1991 19(1):29S.
14. Nagamura-Inoue T, He H. Umbilical cord-derived mesenchymal stem cells: Their advantages and potential clinical utility. *World Journal of Stem Cells.* 2014 6(2):195–202.
15. Jeong JA, Hong SH et al. Differential gene expression profiling of human umbilical cord blood–derived mesenchymal stem cells by DNA microarray. *Stem Cells.* 2005 23(4):584–593.
16. Lee OK, Kuo TK et al. Isolation of multipotent mesenchymal stem cells from umbilical cord blood. *Blood.* 2004 103(5):1669–1675.
17. Kang X-Q, Zang W-J et al. Differentiating characterization of human umbilical cord blood-derived mesenchymal stem cells in vitro. *Cell Biology International.* 2006 30(7):569–575.
18. D'Ippolito G, Schiller PC et al. Age-related osteogenic potential of mesenchymal stromal stem cells from human vertebral bone marrow. *Journal of Bone and Mineral Research.* 1999 14(7):1115–1122.
19. Oreffo ROC, Bord S et al. Skeletal progenitor cells and ageing human populations. *Clinical Science.* 1998 94(5):549–555.
20. Levi BP, Morrison SJ. Stem cells use distinct self-renewal programs at different ages. *Cold Spring Harbor Symposia on Quantitative Biology.* 2008 73:539–553.
21. De Coppi P, Bartsch Jr G et al. Isolation of amniotic stem cell lines with potential for therapy. *Nature Biotechnology.* 2007 25(1):100–106.
22. Karlsson H, Erkers T et al. Stromal cells from term fetal membrane are highly suppressive in allogeneic settings in vitro. *Clinical & Experimental Immunology.* 2012 167(3):543–555.
23. Wolbank S, van Griensven M et al. Alternative sources of adult stem cells: Human amniotic membrane. In: Kasper C, van Griensven M, Pörtner R (Eds.). *Bioreactor Systems for Tissue Engineering II: Strategies for the Expansion and Directed Differentiation of Stem Cells.* Berlin, Germany: Springer; 2010. pp. 1–27.
24. Chen J, Shehadah A et al. Neuroprotective effect of human placenta-derived cell treatment of stroke in rats. *Cell Transplantion.* 2013 22(5):871–879.

25. Kim K-S, Kim HS et al. Long-term immunomodulatory effect of amniotic stem cells in an Alzheimer's disease model. *Neurobiology of Aging*. 2013 34(10):2408–2820.
26. Lee HJ, Jung J et al. Comparison of in vitro hepatogenic differentiation potential between various placenta-derived stem cells and other adult stem cells as an alternative source of functional hepatocytes. *Differentiation*. 2012 84(3):223–231.
27. Chang C-M, Kao C-L et al. Placenta-derived multipotent stem cells induced to differentiate into insulin-positive cells. *Biochemical and Biophysical Research Communications*. 2007 357(2):414–420.
28. Kadam S, Muthyala S et al. Human placenta-derived mesenchymal stem cells and islet-like cell clusters generated from these cells as a novel source for stem cell therapy in diabetes. *The Review of Diabetic Studies: RDS*. 2010 7(2):168–182.
29. Cargnoni A, Di Marcello M et al. Amniotic membrane patching promotes ischemic rat heart repair. *Cell Transplantation*. 2009 18(10–11):1147–1159.
30. Chambers DC, Enever D et al. A phase 1b study of placenta-derived mesenchymal stromal cells in patients with idiopathic pulmonary fibrosis. *Respirology*. 2014 19(7):1013–1018.
31. Jones GN, Moschidou D et al. Potential of human fetal chorionic stem cells for the treatment of osteogenesis imperfecta. *Stem Cells and Development*. 2014 23(3):262–276.
32. Gimble JM, Katz AJ et al. Adipose-derived stem cells for regenerative medicine. *Circulation Research*. 2007 100(9):1249–1260.
33. Nambu M, Kishimoto S et al. Accelerated wound healing in healing-impaired db/db mice by autologous adipose tissue-derived stromal cells combined with atelocollagen matrix. *Annals of Plastic Surgery*. 2009 62(3):317–321.
34. Rigotti G, Marchi A et al. Clinical treatment of radiotherapy tissue damage by lipoaspirate transplant: A healing process mediated by adipose-derived adult stem cells. *Plastic and Reconstructive Surgery*. 2007 119(5):1409–1422.
35. Kyu-Sup C, Hwan-Jung R. Immunomodulatory effects of adipose-derived stem cells in airway allergic diseases. *Current Stem Cell Research & Therapy*. 2010 5(2):111–115.
36. Alperovich M, Lee Z-H et al. Adipose stem cell therapy in cancer reconstruction: A critical review. *Annals of Plastic Surgery*. 2014 73(Suppl 1):S104–S107.
37. Buttery, Bourne S et al. Differentiation of osteoblasts and in vitro bone formation from murine embryonic stem cells. *Tissue Engineering*. 2001 7(1):89–99.
38. Sottile V, Thomson A et al. In vitro osteogenic differentiation of human ES cells. *Cloning & Stem Cells*. 2003 5(2):149–155.
39. Wobus AM, Boheler KR. Embryonic stem cells: Prospects for developmental biology and cell therapy. *Physiological Reviews*. 2005 85(2):635–678.
40. Piltti KM, Salazar DL et al. Safety of human neural stem cell transplantation in chronic spinal cord injury. *Stem Cells Translational Medicine*. 2013 2(12):961–974.
41. Ilic D, Devito L et al. Human embryonic and induced pluripotent stem cells in clinical trials. *British Medical Bulletin*. 2015 116(1):19–27.
42. Schwartz SD, Hubschman J-P et al. Embryonic stem cell trials for macular degeneration: A preliminary report. *The Lancet*. 2012 379(9817):713–720.
43. Takahashi K, Yamanaka S. Induction of pluripotent stem cells from mouse embryonic and adult fibroblast cultures by defined factors. *Cell*. 2006 126(4):663–676.
44. Takahashi K, Tanabe K et al. Induction of pluripotent stem cells from adult human fibroblasts by defined factors. *Cell*. 2007 131(5):861–872.
45. Serra M, Brito C et al. Process engineering of human pluripotent stem cells for clinical application. *Trends in Biotechnology*. 2012 30(6):350–359.
46. Stewart MH, Bosse M et al. Clonal isolation of hESCs reveals heterogeneity within the pluripotent stem cell compartment. *Nature Methods*. 2006 3(10):807–815.
47. Liang G, Zhang Y. Genetic and epigenetic variations in iPSCs: Potential causes and implications for application. *Cell Stem Cell*. 2013 13(2):149–159.

48. Lee AS, Tang C et al. Tumorigenicity as a clinical hurdle for pluripotent stem cell therapies. *Nature Medicine*. 2013 19(8):998–1004.

49. Malchenko S, Galat V et al. Cancer hallmarks in induced pluripotent cells: New insights. *Journal of Cellular Physiology*. 2010 225(2):390–393.

50. Thomson JA, Itskovitz-Eldor J et al. Embryonic stem cell lines derived from human blastocysts. *Science*. 1998 282(5391):1145–1147.

51. Genbacev O, Krtolica A et al. Serum-free derivation of human embryonic stem cell lines on human placental fibroblast feeders. *Fertility and Sterility*. 2005 83(5):1517–15129.

52. Li Y, Powell S et al. Expansion of human embryonic stem cells in defined serum-free medium devoid of animal-derived products. *Biotechnology and Bioengineering*. 2005 91(6):688–698.

53. Braam SR, Zeinstra L et al. Recombinant vitronectin is a functionally defined substrate that supports human embryonic stem cell self-renewal via αVβ5 integrin. *Stem Cells*. 2008 26(9):2257–2265.

54. Sotiropoulou PA, Perez SA et al. Characterization of the optimal culture conditions for clinical scale production of human mesenchymal stem cells. *Stem Cells*. 2006 24(2):462471.

55. Müller I, Kordowich S et al. Application of multipotent mesenchymal stromal cells in pediatric patients following allogeneic stem cell transplantation. *Blood Cells, Molecules, and Diseases*. 2008 40(1):25–32.

56. Prasad VK, Lucas KG et al. Efficacy and safety of ex vivo cultured adult human mesenchymal stem cells (Prochymal™) in pediatric patients with severe refractory acute graft-versus-host disease in a compassionate use study. *Biology of Blood and Marrow Transplantation*. 2011 17(4):534–541.

57. Kebriaei P, Isola L et al. Adult human mesenchymal stem cells added to corticosteroid therapy for the treatment of acute graft-versus-host disease. *Biology of Blood and Marrow Transplantation*. 2009 15(7):804–811.

58. Le Blanc K, Frassoni F et al. Mesenchymal stem cells for treatment of steroid-resistant, severe, acute graft-versus-host disease: A phase II study. *The Lancet*. 2008 371(9624):1579–1586.

59. Wu K-H, Chan C-K et al. Effective treatment of severe steroid-resistant acute graft-versus-host disease with umbilical cord-derived mesenchymal stem cells. *Transplantation*. 2011 91(12):1412–1416.

60. Choi MR, Kim HY et al. Selection of optimal passage of bone marrow-derived mesenchymal stem cells for stem cell therapy in patients with amyotrophic lateral sclerosis. *Neuroscience Letters*. 2010 472(2):94–98.

61. Connick P, Kolappan M et al. The mesenchymal stem cells in multiple sclerosis (MSCIMS) trial protocol and baseline cohort characteristics: An open-label pre-test: Post-test study with blinded outcome assessments. *Trials*. 2011 12:62.

62. Karussis D, Karageorgiou C et al. Safety and immunological effects of mesenchymal stem cell transplantation in patients with multiple sclerosis and amyotrophic lateral sclerosis. *Archives of Neurology*. 2010 67(10):1187–1194.

63. Han Z, Jing Y et al. The role of immunosuppression of mesenchymal stem cells in tissue repair and tumor growth. *Cell & Bioscience*. 2012 2:8.

64. Uccelli A, Moretta L et al. Mesenchymal stem cells in health and disease. *Nature Reviews Immunology*. 2008 8(9):726–736.

65. Krishnamurthy R, Manning MC. The stability factor: Importance in formulation development. *Current Pharmaceutical Biotechnology*. 2002 3(4):361–371.

66. Cross M, Dexter TM. Growth factors in development, transformation, and tumorigenesis. *Cell*. 1991 64(2):271–280.

67. Cohen GB, Ren R et al. Modular binding domains in signal transduction proteins. Cell. 1995 80(2):237–248.

68. Carmeliet P. Angiogenesis in health and disease. *Nature Medicine*. 2003 9(6):653–660.

69. Lanza RP, Langer R et al. *Principles of Tissue Engineering.* Amsterdam, the Netherlands: Elsevier Academic Press; 2007.

70. Dawson E, Mapili G et al. Biomaterials for stem cell differentiation. *Advanced Drug Delivery Reviews.* 2008 60(2):215–228.

71. Lutolf MP, Hubbell JA. Synthetic biomaterials as instructive extracellular microenvironments for morphogenesis in tissue engineering. *Nature Biotechnology.* 2005 23(1):47–55.

72. Davis I, Morstyn G. Clinical uses of growth factors. *Ballière's Clinical Haematology.* 2011 5(3):753–786.

73. Hoffman DI, Zellman GL et al. Cryopreserved embryos in the United States and their availability for research. *Fertility and Sterility.* 2003 79(5):1063–1069.

74. Howard D, Buttery LD et al. Tissue engineering: Strategies, stem cells and scaffolds. *Journal of Anatomy.* 2008 213(1):66–72.

75. Hipp J, Atala A. Tissue engineering, stem cells, cloning, and parthenogenesis: New paradigms for therapy. *Journal of Experimental & Clinical Assisted Reproduction.* 2004 1:3.

76. Colman A, Kind A. Therapeutic cloning: Concepts and practicalities. *Trends in Biotechnology.* 2000 18(5):192–196.

77. Vogelstein B, Alberts B et al. Please don't call it cloning! *Science.* 2002 295(5558):1237.

78. Hochedlinger K, Jaenisch R. Nuclear transplantation, embryonic stem cells, and the potential for cell therapy. *New England Journal of Medicine.* 2003 349(3):275–286.

79. Lanza RP, Cibelli JB et al. The ethical reasons for stem cell research. *Science.* 2001 292(5520):1299.

80. Lanza RP, Cibelli JB et al. Prospects for the use of nuclear transfer in human transplantation. *Nature Biotechnology.* 1999 17(12):1171–1174.

81. Klimanskaya I, Hipp J et al. Derivation and comparative assessment of retinal pigment epithelium from human embryonic stem cells using transcriptomics. *Cloning and Stem Cells.* 2004 6(3):217–245.

82. Mehedintu M, Berg H. Proliferation response of yeast saccharomyces cerevisiae on electromagnetic field parameters. *Bioelectrochemistry and Bioenergetics.* 1997 43(1):67–70.

83. Smith SD, McLeod BR et al. Calcium cyclotron resonance and diatom mobility. *Bioelectromagnetics.* 1987 8(3):215–227.

84. Garcia AM, Frank EH et al. Contributions of fluid convection and electrical migration to transport in cartilage: Relevance to loading. *Archives of Biochemistry and Biophysics.* 1996 333(2):317–325.

85. Grodzinsky AJ, Frank EH. Cartilage electromechanics–I. Electrokinetic transduction and the effects of electrolyte pH and ionic strength. *Journal of Biomechanical Engineering.* 1987 20(6):615–627.

86. Kim Y-J, Bonassar LJ et al. The role of cartilage streaming potential, fluid flow and pressure in the stimulation of chondrocyte biosynthesis during dynamic compression. *Journal of Biomechanics.* 1995 28(9):1055–1066.

87. Fan G-C. Role of heat shock proteins in stem cell behavior. *Progress in Molecular Biology and Translational Science.* 2012 111:305–322.

88. Chao E, Inoue N. Biophysical stimulation of bone fracture repair, regeneration and remodelling. *European Cells & Materials.* 2003 6:72–84.

89. Wiesmann HP, Joos U et al. Biological and biophysical principles in extracorporal bone tissue engineering. Part II. *International Journal of Oral and Maxillofacial Surgery.* 2004 33(6):523–530.

90. Barrère F, Mahmood TA et al. Advanced biomaterials for skeletal tissue regeneration: Instructive and smart functions. *Materials Science and Engineering: R: Reports.* 2008 59(1–6):38–71.

91. Dimitriou R, Babis GC. Biomaterial osseointegration enhancement with biophysical stimulation. *Journal of Musculoskeletal and Neuronal Interactions.* 2007 7(3):253–265.

92. Olkku A, Leskinen JJ et al. Ultrasound-induced activation of Wnt signaling in human MG-63 osteoblastic cells. *Bone.* 47(2):320–330.

93. Lin F-H, Lin C-C et al. The effects of ultrasonic stimulation on DP-bioglass bone substitute. *Medical Engineering Physics*. 1995 17(1):20–26.
94. Tanzer M, Harvey E et al. Effect of noninvasive low intensity ultrasound on bone growth into porous-coated implants. *Journal of Orthopaedic Research*. 1996 14(6):901–906.
95. Tsai M-T, Chang WH-S et al. Pulsed electromagnetic fields affect osteoblast proliferation and differentiation in bone tissue engineering. *Bioelectromagnetics*. 2007 28(7):519–528.
96. Hernández-Bule ML, Roldán E et al. Radiofrequency currents exert cytotoxic effects in NB69 human neuroblastoma cells but not in peripheral blood mononuclear cells. *International Journal of Oncology*. 2012 41(4):1251–1259.
97. Hernández-Bule ML, Trillo MÁ et al. Molecular mechanisms underlying antiproliferative and differentiating responses of hepatocarcinoma cells to subthermal electric stimulation. *PLoS One*. 2014 9(1):e84636.
98. Gardner S, Frantz R et al. Effect of electrical stimulation on chronic wound healing: A meta-analysis. *Wound Repair and Regeneration*. 1999 7(6):495–503.
99. Recio AC, Felter CE et al. High-voltage electrical stimulation for the management of stage III and IV pressure ulcers among adults with spinal cord injury: Demonstration of its utility for recalcitrant wounds below the level of injury. *The Journal of Spinal Cord Medicine*. 2012 35(1):58–63.
100. Young S, Hampton S et al. Study to evaluate the effect of low-intensity pulsed electrical currents on levels of oedema in chronic non-healing wounds. *Journal of Wound Care*. 2011 20(8):368–373.
101. Sun S, Titushkin I et al. Regulation of mesenchymal stem cell adhesion and orientation in 3D collagen scaffold by electrical stimulus. *Bioelectrochemistry*. 2006 69(2):133–141.
102. Tandon N, Goh B et al. Alignment and elongation of human adipose-derived stem cells in response to direct-current electrical stimulation. *Conference proceedings: Annual International Conference of the IEEE Engineering in Medicine and Biology Society IEEE Engineering in Medicine and Biology Society Conference*. 2009 1:6517–6521.
103. Hernández-Bule ML CM, Trillo MA, Leal J, Ubeda A. Cytostatic response of HepG2 to 0.57 MHz electric currents mediated by changes in cell cycle control proteins. *International Journal of Oncology*. 2010 37(6):1399–1405.
104. Hernández-Bule, Paíno CL et al. Electric stimulation at 448 kHz promotes proliferation of human mesenchymal stem cells. *Cellular Physiology and Biochemistry*. 2014 34(5):1741–1755.
105. Sun, Hsieh D-K et al. Effect of pulsed electromagnetic field on the proliferation and differentiation potential of human bone marrow mesenchymal stem cells. *Bioelectromagnetics*. 2009 30(4):251–260.
106. Zhong C, Zhang X et al. Effects of low-intensity electromagnetic fields on the proliferation and differentiation of cultured mouse bone marrow stromal cells. *Physical Therapy*. 2012 92(9):1208–1219.
107. Li X, Zhang M et al. Effects of 50 Hz pulsed electromagnetic fields on the growth and cell cycle arrest of mesenchymal stem cells: An in vitro study. *Electromagnetic Biology and Medicine*. 2012 31(4):356–364.
108. Hardy, RC, Sukhavasi et al. Electrical stimulation of human mesenchymal stem cells on biomineralized conducting polymers enhances their differentiation towards osteogenic outcomes. *Journal of Materials Chemistry*. 2015 3(41):8059–8064.
109. Ahn H-J, Lee W-J et al. FGF2 stimulates the proliferation of human mesenchymal stem cells through the transient activation of JNK signaling. *FEBS Letters*. 2009 583(17):2922–2926.
110. Hanada K, Dennis JE et al. Stimulatory effects of basic fibroblast growth factor and bone morphogenetic protein-2 on osteogenic differentiation of rat bone marrow-derived mesenchymal stem cells. *Journal of Bone and Mineral Research*. 1997 12(10):1606–1614.
111. Gesta S, Tseng Y-H et al. Developmental origin of fat: Tracking obesity to its source. *Cell*. 2007 131(2):242–256.

112. Liu H, Fergusson MM et al. Augmented Wnt signaling in a mammalian model of accelerated aging. *Science*. 2007 317(5839):803–806.
113. Astudillo P, Ríos S et al. Increased adipogenesis of osteoporotic human-mesenchymal stem cells (MSCs) characterizes by impaired leptin action. *Journal of Cellular Biochemistry*. 2008 103(4):1054–1065.
114. Uda Y, Poh Y-C et al. Force via integrins but not E-cadherin decreases Oct3/4 expression in embryonic stem cells. *Biochemical and Biophysical Research Communications*. 2011 415(2):396–400.
115. Takahashi, Nuckolls GH et al. Compressive force promotes sox9, type II collagen and aggrecan and inhibits IL-1beta expression resulting in chondrogenesis in mouse embryonic limb bud mesenchymal cells. *Journal of Cell Science*. 1998 111(14):2067–2076.
116. Kang, Yoon H-H et al. Effect of mechanical stimulation on the differentiation of cord stem cells. *Connective Tissue Research*. 2012 53(2):149–159.
117. Kearney EM, Farrell E et al. Tensile strain as a regulator of mesenchymal stem cell osteogenesis. *Annals of Biomedical Engineering*. 2010 38(5):1767–1779.
118. Chen J, Li C et al. Periodic heat shock accelerated the chondrogenic differentiation of human mesenchymal stem cells in pellet culture. *PLoS One*. 2014 9(3):e91561.
119. Chen J, Shi ZD et al. Enhanced osteogenesis of human mesenchymal stem cells by periodic heat shock in self-assembling peptide hydrogel. *Tissue Engineering Part A*. 2013 19(5–6):716–728.
120. Doyle J, Smart B. Stimulation of bone growth by short-wave diathermy. *Journal of Bone and Joint Surgery American*. 1963 45(1):15–24.
121. Richards V, Stofer R. The stimulation of bone growth by internal heating. *Annals of Surgery*. 1959 46(1):84–96.
122. Kern B, Shen J et al. Cbfa1 contributes to the osteoblast-specific expression of type I collagen genes. *The Journal of Biological Chemistry*. 2001 276(10):7101–7107.

Index

Note: Page numbers in bold and italics refer to tables and figures, respectively.

Printed and bound by CPI Group (UK) Ltd, Croydon, CR0 4YY

17/10/2024

01775663-0003